Kathryn Marsden's
Super Skin

ABOUT THE AUTHOR

Kathryn was born in 1951 and brought up in a small village in the North Cotswold Hills. She trained and qualified in hotel management which sparked her all-consuming interest in nutrition and food science. When her husband Ralph was diagnosed with cancer, she embarked upon an ambitious study of different dietary treatments which might help him. She became so enthralled by the fascinating potential of simple food substances in treating disease that she turned her attention full-time to the health, beauty and fitness field.

Kathryn went on to study physiology, anatomy, biology, biochemistry and the naturopathic and orthomolecular approaches to nutrition. She holds a Diploma in Clinical Nutrition and Nutritional Counselling and maintains up-to-the-minute research into scientific studies and reviews of new nutritional methods worldwide.

Apart from a hectic schedule of writing, teaching and media work, she continues to run a busy practice dealing with requests for help from people with a diverse number of illnesses. It is her experiences in treating a wide range of skin conditions that led to the writing of *Kathryn Marsden's Super Skin*. Also a freelance journalist and columnist, she writes regularly for many women's magazines, the health press and journals. Kathryn's is a familiar voice on BBC, local and independent radio and television. She is a member of the Faculty of the The Tisserand Institute and teaches nutrition to students at the Royal Masonic Hospital and at Colleges of Further Education. Much in demand as an after dinner speaker, she gives lectures and seminars worldwide.

Kathryn is author of the best seller *The Food Combining Diet* which has helped thousands of people to lose weight safely and successfully without cutting calories.

Kathryn Marsden's
Super Skin

Thorsons
An Imprint of HarperCollinsPublishers

This book is dedicated to Vicki Dryden Wyatt, Marion Richards, Rachel Carse, Kate Histed and everyone at The PR Workshop for their never-failing kindness, concern and guidance.

Thorsons
An Imprint of HarperCollins*Publishers*
77–85 Fulham Palace Road
Hammersmith, London W6 8JB

First published by Thorsons 1993
This edition 1996
10 9 8 7 6 5 4 3 2

© Kathryn Marsden 1993

Kathryn Marsden asserts the moral right to
be identified as the author of this work

A catalogue record for this book
is available from the British Library

ISBN 0 7225 3379 9

Illustrations by Andrea Norton, except drawing on p.110 by Peter Cox

Typeset by Harper Phototypesetters Limited,
Northampton, England
Printed in Great Britain by
Caledonian International Book Manufacturing Ltd, Glasgow

Contents

Acknowledgements

My very grateful thanks go to:

Katie Boyle - for writing the Foreword to *Kathryn Marsden's Super Skin*. I am very touched by her generous words.

Leslie Kenton - for her support and encouragement.

Kathleen Young at Oriflame UK.

Dr John Stirling for, once again, minutely checking the technical details in my manuscript.

My friends - and multi-talented support team! - Annie Runyard RGN, Kathy Webb (hair stylist), Sharon Clarke (beautician) and Maggie Fillingham (aromatherapist).

Ralph, my lovely husband - for editing and printing the manuscript.

Sarah Sutton - for her care and gentle guidance.

Rosemary Staheyeff - for her common sense and her empathetic editing.

There's nothing worth the wear of winning
But laughter and the love of friends.

Hilaire Belloc (1870–1953)

Foreword

After the runaway success of Kathryn Marsden's book *The Food Combining Diet*, I reached out eagerly for her next publication.

I wasn't disappointed. The Marsden Magic was there again: real knowledge of her subject, combined with sensible solutions to the problems she tackles.

I feel so safe in Kathryn Marsden's hands, and her direct style makes her advice very easy to follow.

Katie Boyle

Preface

This book is for anyone who has a skin problem - whether it be dry, oily, flaky, dull, blemished or just in need of care and attention. If you are concerned about wrinkles and ageing or *tempus fugit* (literally, 'time flies'), then this book is for you, too.

Skin problems can make life a misery. I know: I speak from irksome experience. From the onset of periods at age 14, I began my fight against the dreaded zits. 'There, there', 'You'll grow out of it' and sympathetic head-patting from dermatologists, doctors and relatives did absolutely nothing to make me feel better.

Long and arduous visits to a number of hospitals and a variety of different specialists eventually detected a serious endocrine disorder ('probably inherited') which, it was felt, 'might' ('or might not') be causing or aggravating the skin problem. A whole gamut of medical tests resulted in two major operations which eased the hormonal horrors - but the eruptions persisted.

Could it be my diet? 'What you eat will make no difference whatsoever to the condition of your skin', I was (or so I thought) reliably informed. And twenty-five years later, a leaflet to be found in most doctors' waiting rooms continues to maintain that what a person eats will have neither beneficial nor detrimental effect upon their skin condition. 'There is no scientific evidence that chocolate or fatty foods contribute to the problem', it proclaims.

Then it must, I decided, have something to do with what I put on the outside. I turned my attention to lots of pots of lotions and potions but, despite copious and diligent application, these affected only the existing spots and did nothing to prevent new ones from forming. Over-enthusiastic dedication to very strong-smelling chemical astringents made matters much worse, adding dry, sore and flaky skin to the ever-present blemishes and leaving me with red blotches and scarring. Perhaps, after all, I would just have to wait to grow out of it.

On reaching the milestone of 21, I was convinced that I would soon be spot free. No such luck. 'Growing out of it' was obviously not going to happen to me.

But my skin *has* improved enormously – through diet. Its condition now bears no comparison to the angry, sore appearance that I suffered – and tried in vain to hide – for so many years. Because of the previously over-aggressive treatments, it will never be absolutely perfect but, even the deep blemishes, which I was told would always be there, fade a little more with each passing year.

Now, if what the medical establishment says about diet having no effect on the resolution of skin disorders is true, how is it that I – and many others – have managed to attain a good complexion by eating the right kinds of food, using the right skin-care products, following a regular detoxification programme and taking regular exercise?

I have had patients who swear that one piece of chocolate equals one spot and that a high-fat diet definitely aggravates the problem. Well, in my experience as a spot-ridden teenager turned clear-skinned nutritionist, I agree with them. Just show me a box of chocolates and zits appear on the horizon. My only regret is that it took so many years for me to discover that the 'experts' might not have all the answers.

Treating the surface symptoms i.e. the dryness, the blemishes, the eczema etc. is all very well but does nothing to discover or resolve the cause of the condition. And pugnacious attack is, for some indefinable reason, still considered a medical priority. A book on skin care, written by an alleged authority and published as recently as 1992, continues to follow the line that acne should be treated with antibiotics – advice which I find both misleading and alarming.

Long-term ingestion of antibiotics cures nothing, but has the potential for causing a wide range of other illnesses. Experience has shown me that the way to success is to treat the whole body, inside and out, *naturally*. Although they may not be enough on their own, skin-care products are vitally important. Diet is also a significant factor but, without a top-quality cleansing and nourishing routine (externally and internally), may not be so effective. Sensible exercise and de-stressing techniques are also valuable virtues.

If you have a particular skin problem which needs special attention or are still unsure about your skin type, you may benefit from the advice available from the beauty counter consultants who hold court in most of the larger department stores. But talk to as many as possible; it will help you to sort the sales hype from the worthwhile guidance.

Whilst writing and researching this book, I talked to consultants from all the major skin-care and cosmetic companies. I found it confusing that each one offered different advice, which just goes to show that the experts all have individual ideas and views on how to achieve perfect skin, and every person has utterly individual requirements. In the space of one week, I was told I had oily, combination, sensitive, not sensitive and dry skin. I should exfoliate more often; I should exfoliate less often; I should use a special eye cleanser; no, that wasn't necessary as my ordinary cleanser was adequate, etc. etc. I also enjoyed several make-up sessions – although many of the consultants' ideas on which colours suited me were so way off the mark that several friends wondered if I was quite well . . . eye liner and foundation (which I rarely wear), brown and purple shadows, overemphasized blusher and dark lipstick conspired to make a healthy nutritionist look tired and consumptive!

At the end of it all, I was able to take the best bits of advice from all the sources I had consulted and put them together in a package to suit my personal needs. There are lots of great products around which, in my view, make a definite difference to skin health and condition.

If you are unsure, ask for samples to try before you buy and don't be persuaded into purchasing lots of full-sized expensive jars and bottles which may be unsuitable. However helpful your consultant is, she is there to sell her company's products! If you even suspect that you won't use a product, don't be pressurized into buying it. And don't fall for the sales pitch that one product won't work unless it is used in conjunction with another – it's unlikely to be true.

Women's magazines are also a valuable source of information on skin care and make up.

If you are unable, or find it difficult, to leave the house, seek out a home consultant who can advise you and allow you to sample products before buying. (Further details on p.218.)

I have always wanted to write a book about skin to record my own observations so that they might help others. Some of the tips included may not toe the orthodox line but they are gentle, entirely safe and, most important of all, they work.

A list outlining the subjects covered appears at the beginning of each chapter.

I am not a skin specialist or a beautician and would not wish, in any way, to denigrate those professionals. I write purely from my own experience – and that of my patients – through which I hope to show you the natural way to a clear, glowing and healthy complexion.

Kathryn Marsden
Wiltshire, England

P.S. As far as my extensive research can confirm, none of the methods or products mentioned in the book have caused harm to any animal. Animals don't wear cosmetics. Because we do, why should they suffer?

Introduction: The Super Skin Strategy

Beauty of face is a frail ornament, a passing flower, a momentary brightness belonging to the skin.

J.B. Poquelin, pen name Molière (1622–73)

LOOKING GOOD

Appearances do matter. Looking good makes people feel good. Looking after yourself and your skin makes good sense. How you look projects your personality and demonstrates that you are thinking positively about yourself.

For the young, looking good becomes all important – for some a consuming passion. But an acne-ridden teenager or a 25-year old with very dry or very oily skin and lacklustre locks may feel that there is little point in bothering, especially if they have already tried to resolve their problems without success. And for many more, as the years advance, interest in hair care, skin care, make-up, healthy eating, posture and dress begins to wane. It shouldn't have to and doesn't need to. I'm convinced that lots of very lovely people never reach their full potential simply because they hide themselves and their inner beauty underneath shapeless, colourless clothing, dull, lifeless hair, a boring, flavourless and nutrient deficient diet and dated or non-existent make-up. No wonder they feel depressed, tired and lacking in self-esteem.

There are bound to be people reading this who disagree with

me. 'Bah! Humbug!' they will say. It doesn't matter what someone looks like. It's the actual person that is important. Inner beauty will shine through no matter what.

Of course it can. But what's wrong with giving it a little encouragement? After all, how a person looks is often a reflection of how they feel. And feelings affect attitude.

Cosmetic beauty may be only skin deep but real beauty reflects your whole being. And the two *are* connected. I believe that there is an inextricable link between good health and beauty at all levels. Good skin care and hair care can transform a personality. Even something as simple as applying some lipstick or giving your nails a salon treatment can chase a negative outlook away for long enough to spur you into more positive action. Nourishing and nurturing yourself properly brings immense and immeasurable rewards of confidence, vitality, energy, positiveness and good health, of looking and feeling good – inside and out.

And age really has nothing to do with it. One person's wrinkle is merely another person's laughter line.

Kathryn Marsden's Super Skin is full of helpful and healthful beauty tips, advice on diet, hair and nail care, nutritional supplements, first aid for particular problems and how to detoxify and cleanse the system – all designed to get you glowing.

YOUR SKIN AND HOW IT FUNCTIONS

Skin is an amazing structure. The body's largest organ, covering between 15 and 20 square feet (1.5 and 2 square metres), it measures one twentieth of an inch thick and weighs anything from 6 to 9 pounds (2.75 to 4 kilograms). This wonderful 'waterproof' and washable coat serves as a temperature regulator, a major route for the elimination of waste and, given the right nutrients, has the incredible capacity to heal itself when injured and act as an efficient defence against trauma, infection and invasion. 'Like a wax paper that holds everything in without dripping' is how skin was described by the U.S. television personality Art Linkletter.

Healthy skin is slightly acid and is protected by the 'acid mantle', a naturally lubricating mixture of sebum and sweat which provides additional protection against assault by harmful bacteria. The skin and its padding also cushion internal organs against impact.

Through approximately 2,500,000 sweat glands, the average adult human being loses around a pint and a half (850ml) of sweat each day. In every square inch there are hundreds of pain, heat, cold and touch sensors, 15 feet (5 metres) of blood vessels, 12 feet (4 metres) of nerves, 100 sebaceous glands and over 1500 sensory receptors totalling 3 million cells, all shedding constantly – at an amount equal to an entire layer every seven to ten weeks.

This perpetual 'moulting' means that, to maintain the status quo, new cells need to be formed at an equivalent rate.

The outer surface (the epidermis) is actually a layer of dead keratin cells which are continually being shed and replaced by new cells working their way up from the dermis below. When this exfoliation process becomes sluggish – as we grow older or when health is under par – cell renewal slows right down, elimination pathways can become blocked, skin is less supple and so becomes more prone to injury and disease.

To remain in good condition and to work efficiently, your birthday suit needs to be fed and cleaned from the inside as well as the outside.

Kathryn Marsden's Super Skin shows you how.

THE SUPER SKIN STRATEGY

Successful skin care requires a four-pronged protection plan:

1. NUTRITION: A healthy diet brimful of healing and nurturing nutrients

2. PURITY: Internal detoxification and cleansing

3. BEAUTY: External care i.e. deep cleansing, exfoliation, massage, toning and moisturizing

4. WELL-BEING: Relaxation and exercise

Ignoring just one of these important areas is a bit like expecting a four-legged table to stand firmly on only three legs! Without support at all four corners, everything begins to slide and, eventually, crashes to the floor.

Kathryn Marsden's Super Skin shows you how easy it is to achieve a vital visage and confident new countenance by following this simple four-point plan.

ONE

Nutrition

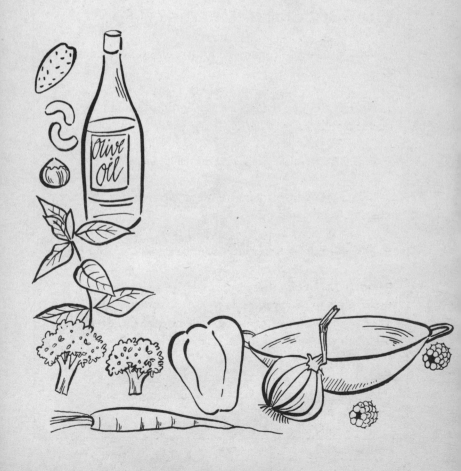

Super Skin Foods –
and Skin Scoundrels

The disease ceases without the use of any kind of medicine, if
only a proper way of living be adopted.

Aetios (c. AD 535)

> Fruit and Vegetables
> Grains
> Sprouted Seeds and Beans
> Herbs
> Garlic
> Olive Oil
> Yoghurt
> Honey and Molasses
> Nuts
> Skin Scoundrels

Everything you (do or don't) put in your mouth is likely to
affect the quality of your skin.

A clogged, spotty complexion often betrays a diet high in fats
and sugars, a history of constipation, kidneys that are not
working at their best or poor lymphatic drainage; an ultra-
sensitive skin may be the result of poor digestion and
inadequate absorption; very dry, flaky skin may indicate deficiencies of essential fatty acids and vitamin E; whilst skin that
refuses to heal could be in need of vitamins A, B_6, C and zinc.

The amazing thing is that skins like these can be completely
transformed by making simple but beneficial changes to the
diet, eating foods in the right combinations, using a regular

internal and external cleansing programme, taking the right supplements and making time for regular exercise.

Skin quality can also be affected by the external environment – by cigarette smoking (passive or direct), traffic fumes, malfunctioning air conditioning systems, central heating, radiation, VDU screens (see p.184) and excessive sun exposure. Nourishing food and protective skin care can help here too, providing defence against infection, cell damage and premature ageing.

The right kinds of foods will keep your intestines free of clutter, encourage all your elimination processes to function efficiently and keep your blood clean and fed with nutrients.

As if put there to increase our anguish, there will always be the gorgeous creature who seems to live on junk food and yet looks wonderful without any apparent effort – probably blessed with an amazingly efficient digestive and detox system which can handle all that rubbish.

For those of us who don't fall into this category, Nature's natural beauty foods are there to help us.

SUPER SKIN FOODS

In their raw state, vegetables, fruits, sprouted grains, sprouted seeds and herbs are rich in nutrients and natural enzymes, so it is important to make sure that your diet contains at least some raw food every day. Many kinds of fresh fruits, vegetables, salads and herbs are sensational skin fixers. They help to renew and refurbish, providing protection against further damage. For example, lemon juice applied topically is cleansing and healing; taken as a drink or in food, it clears and cleanses from the inside out. Grapes, fresh pineapple, apples and kiwi fruits are wonderful skin foods. So are cabbage and vitamin A-rich carrots, beetroot and parsley. Botanicals such as artichoke, burdock, chelidonium, dandelion and sarsaparilla help to decongest the kidneys and liver, improving the outflow of waste products and taking the detox load off the overworked skin.

For the benefit of your skin - and your health - make full use of the healing sustenance provided by Mother Nature. All fruits and vegetables will be of value; so are wholegrains, nuts, seeds, yoghurt, fresh fish - and fresh water! The skin foods detailed here are just some of the very best.

Fruits

Apples
Rich in pectin and vitamin C, essential in any detoxification and skin healing programme and useful for helping to stabilize cholesterol. The tartaric acid and malic acid content of apples helps to settle the digestion. To treat an upset stomach or diarrhoea, grate an apple and leave it exposed to the air for 15 minutes before eating. It seems that this is one of those rare instances where oxidation (browning) is therapeutic. Don't do this to fruit as a general rule, though! When slicing or grating apples for other purposes, always have fresh lemon juice handy to sprinkle over them - the lemon stops the apple from going brown. Apples are an excellent health tonic for the bowel and liver and apple juice a helpful remedy for the treatment of kidney stones and gallstones. Unfortunately, many fruit crops

have become victims of over-zealous pesticide use so, unless you know they are organic, it's best to discard the skins.

Apricots

Fresh or dried, apricots are loaded with beta-carotene and iron, both important skin nutrients. An excellent cleansing fruit. At times of illness – especially bronchitis, chest and throat infections, colds, catarrh or sinusitis – use a juicing machine or food processor to blend apricots into a soothing and nourishing drink. They are also reported to be beneficial in the treatment of constipation, intestinal parasites and gallstones. Try the familiar dried yellow apricots or the hard, round Hunza apricots. Washed thoroughly and soaked overnight, they make a wonderfully nourishing and sustaining start to the day. But avoid those that are sprayed with sulphur dioxide preservative and glazing agents: sulphites can cause skin rashes.

Bananas

I read recently that bananas should not be included in any cleansing diet because of their starch content. In fact, they are a rich source of potassium, vitamin A, vitamin C, iron, calcium, zinc, folic acid and pectin – all essential for healthy skin. Bananas are high in gentle but effective dietary fibre and are an excellent therapeutic for all kinds of bowel disorders – particularly constipation, haemorrhoids, colitis, irritable bowel and diarrhoea. An average-sized banana contains only 90 Calories but is filling, sustaining and easy on the digestion – very useful as an energy boost between meals and especially helpful if you are trying to overcome 'chocoholism'. I see no reason whatsoever to *exclude* them.

Blackberries

A rich source of vitamin C. Very valuable as a blood cleansing food, blackberries are recommended for the treatment of excess mucus - in catarrh, for example - and for constipation, anaemia, kidney problems, diarrhoea and menstrual cramps. An infusion made from blackberry leaves is wonderfully therapeutic for sore throats.

Blueberries
Well known for their antiseptic and blood cleansing properties, blueberries can be helpful for anaemia, bowel problems, spots and blemishes and menstrual disorders. A good source of vitamins and minerals.

Figs
Fresh or dried, figs are packed with nourishment. Rich in calcium, iron and magnesium, dried figs are also one of the best fibre sources. Six dried figs and three glasses of water added daily to the diet is an excellent remedy for constipation. A sluggish bowel can be a common companion to a sallow or spotty skin! Figs are also reported to be helpful in the treatment of Raynaud's syndrome, poor circulation, hypotension (low blood pressure), intestinal parasites and catarrh. The juice from soaked figs makes an excellent cough medicine and gargle for sore throats. Split open and soaked for five minutes in hand-hot water, fresh figs make a soothing poultice for boils and for abscesses of the skin or gums.

Grapefruit
Valuable for its fibre, pectin and vitamin C. The bioflavonoids, found in the pith and skin segments, are blood vessel strengtheners, anti-inflammatory agents, powerful antioxidants and fighters of infection - all vital in the quest for healthy skin. An interesting point which I have noted with my own patients is that whereas oranges and orange juice can aggravate

arthritic conditions, fresh grapefruit seems to be helpful. Save grapefruit skin, grate and dry it and store in an airtight container; during the winter, use a teaspoon of the rind with equal quantities of mint, sage and dark honey as a soothing cold remedy.

Grapes

Eat as many as you like. Why not have a 'grape day' and eat nothing else. You'll munch your way through 3lb (1.5kg) or more but shouldn't feel hungry. You'll rest your digestion, speed up the detox process and help your skin – all at the same time. Make sure that you wash the grapes really thoroughly. Drink plenty of filtered or spring water throughout the day, too, around 3 pints (1.7 litres).

Kiwi Fruit

Contain twice the vitamin C of an orange, around four times the fibre of a stick of celery and are a good source of vitamin E and potassium. A versatile fruit, wonderful for juicing and for packed lunches. Just cut in half and scoop the flesh from the skin with a teaspoon or peel and slice.

Lemons

One of life's greatest cleansers, packed with vitamin C (twice that of oranges) *and* they contain those valuable bioflavonoids. Lemons are one of the top skin foods, cleansing, healing and protective of the delicate mucous membranes – the body's 'inside skin'. Wake up to a drink of hot water with a squeeze of fresh lemon juice. If you find the taste too sharp, then add a dribble of organic honey. Use boiled water, though, not water from the hot tap. And remember that lemon juice sold in bottles or plastic imitation lemons will contain preservative. An old remedy for wrinkles was to apply lemon juice directly to the skin, leave it for two or three hours and then massage with olive oil; this is also beneficial for the hands. A lemon juice and water rinse is good for dandruff and makes a cleansing mouthwash - especially helpful after a late night or an excess of alcohol when the inside of the mouth and throat feels 'unpleasant'. Rub lemon juice into the hands to remove stains, to heal cuts and to eliminate the odour of onions or fish.

Melons

It was once believed that melons were a waste of time from a nutritional point of view because they were nearly 90 per cent water. Now we know that all melons are nourishing and cleansing, rich in vitamin C and potassium and a good source of folic acid, vitamin A and iron. Cantaloup and watermelon are particularly valuable. Melons prefer to be eaten entirely on their own, not with any other kind of food: mixing them causes fermentation, digestive distress and poor absorption of nutrients. If you eat them as a starter, try to leave 15 minutes between courses.

Pineapple

Fresh pineapple contains some very useful enzymes and lots of vitamins and minerals; it's particularly rich in vitamin C and bromelain, both of which have anti-inflammatory properties. The heavier the pineapple, the more juice it is likely to contain. Canned pineapple (in its own juice) can be a useful standby but is far less nourishing than the fresh version.

Pumpkin

A very rich source of beta carotene, pumpkin makes a versatile addition to both sweet and savoury dishes. Reported to be beneficial in the treatment of fluid retention, low blood pressure, inflammation, ulceration, piles and varicose veins.

Pumpkin seeds are an excellent skin food, being rich in essential fatty acids. Also good for constipation and, when the seeds are made into a tea, for the elimination of intestinal parasites.

Follow the Fruit Rule
To obtain the maximum nutrient value from your fruit, enjoy it as a between-meal snack, an early morning juice or at the beginning of a meal – in other words, always on an empty stomach. And avoid the common practice of eating an apple or fruit salad as a dessert. Piling the fruit – which requires a fast transit through the digestive system – on top of slow-moving protein or starch means that nothing will be broken down properly; fermentation and incomplete digestion will lead to bloating, flatulence, heartburn and abdominal discomfort.

With the exception of melon, which likes to be eaten entirely separately, all other fruits will mix happily with each other as long as there are no proteins or starches present. So enjoy a mixed fruit salad – but on its own.

Vegetables, Salad Foods and Sprouts

Artichokes
Globe artichokes are a valuable source of calcium, iron, vitamin C, thiamin, niacin and dietary fibre. They have powerful diuretic properties, good for cleaning the liver and the kidneys which, in turn, helps the skin.

Asparagus
Another good internal cleanser, an excellent kidney tonic and a worthwhile source of vitamins C and E. Said to be good for

all kinds of rheumatic and arthritic ailments. Fresh asparagus has such a short season so make use of it when it is around, either steamed and served with a little melted butter or cold in salads with extra virgin olive oil. Asparagus is one of the few acid-forming vegetables (most are alkaline-forming) but it's nourishing nonetheless. And don't be alarmed if your urine smells slightly different on the day or day after you have eaten asparagus; its acid-forming nature alters the odour but this is not believed to be detrimental in any way.

Avocado

Really a fruit but used most often with salads and in savoury dishes, avocados are skin savers in more ways than one. Easy to digest and rich in vitamins A, C, E, some B vitamins and potassium, they also contain monounsaturated fat (see p.49), now known to be beneficial in the war against the bad (LDL) cholesterol (see p.50). Good for ulcers and inflammation of the mucous membrane. Don't avoid avocados if you are trying to cut calories: half an avocado with an olive oil and cider vinegar dressing is a filling, nourishing and sustaining snack at only 200 calories. Avocados also make wonderful skin treatments and are used widely in cosmetic and skin-care products. For a soothing face pack, mash one quarter of a fresh avocado with a dessertspoonful of plain bio-yoghurt. Spread the mixture evenly over the face and neck and leave in place for 15 minutes. Rinse away with tepid water. To make a great hair conditioner, mix and mash half an avocado with a teaspoon of dark liquid honey and two teaspoons of extra virgin olive oil.

Bamboo Shoots

Tender bamboo shoots can be eaten either raw or cooked in boiling water for about ten minutes. They contain vitamins A and C, small amounts of some B vitamins, calcium and iron. A valuable skin food because of their detoxifying talents. Also reported to be beneficial for bowel disorders and high blood pressure.

Barley

Highly regarded as a nutritious food, barley has been used in the treatment of diarrhoea and ulcers, cystitis and fever. It is known to strengthen the hair and nails. It may also be valuable for asthmatics since it contains a substance, hordenine, which relieves bronchial spasm.

Beetroot

The blood builder, a wonderful liver, kidney and bladder tonic and especially beneficial when juiced with apples, carrots and grapes. Raw beetroot is a rich source of iron, vitamin A, vitamin C and calcium and contains other valuable nutrients which are excellent for healthy skin, for strengthening blood vessels, fighting infection, for anaemia and heavy periods. Adding grapes to beetroot juice or beetroot salad is said to improve the absorption of the its nutrients. The strong colouring of urine and faeces caused by beetroot can be alarming but is, in fact, thought to be beneficial to the bowel, kidneys and bladder and not at all dangerous. Avoid pre-cooked beetroot, which usually contains preservatives.

Broccoli

Now known to contain a special anti-cancer chemical called sulphoraphane, broccoli is also a fund of vitamins and minerals including beta carotene, calcium, iron, folic acid and vitamins C and E. A wonderful vegetable for steaming or stir-frying and delicious in salads too.

Cabbage

Lightly steamed or shredded raw cabbage is a vital skin saver. Cabbage water is a useful aid to digestion and a liver system and blood cleanser, making it an important skin food. Also reputed to be good for the hair, nails, teeth, gums and bones. Take care when cooking cabbage; its nutrients, particularly the valuable vitamin C content, are destroyed by prolonged cooking. Finely sliced raw cabbage is wonderful in coleslaw with grated apple, carrot, celery and onion.

Carrot

Carrots are high in fibre, vitamin C and beta carotene, the vegetable form of vitamin A. Great grated raw in salads, juiced, stir-fried, sliced for stews and casseroles or lightly steamed. The antioxidant properties of carrots are vital for healthy blood cells and healthy skin.

Celery and Celeriac

Celery is the stick-shaped stalks that grow out of the celeriac – the celery root. Both are very nourishing, good in all kinds of hot and cold dishes, soups, stews, stir-fries and salads. The celeriac has more fibre than the celery stalks and is slightly richer in vitamin C. The green celery leaves are also good for you; shred them for salads or use for stocks and casseroles. Both celery and celeriac are good kidney cleansers. All parts of the plant (and particularly the seeds) have long been recognized for their therapeutic value to arthritis sufferers.

Chicory

Also known as Belgian endive or witloof. A super skin food with excellent cleansing properties. A tasty addition to salads and particularly enjoyable with apple and avocado. Curly endive is the green relative, a useful source of vitamin C, iron and beta carotene.

Cucumber

This ancient plant of the marrow and pumpkin family is
believed to have been first cultivated in Burma or India around
11,000 years ago. Cucumber extracts can be found in many
cosmetic and skin-care products, particularly toners and
cleansers, and it is easy to make your own preparations at
home. Grate about a quarter of one whole cucumber and
squeeze the juice into half a cupful of milk. Soak cotton pads
with the mixture and use it as a cleanser. It suits all skin
types. Cut slices of cucumber to pep up tired, gritty eyes and
use cucumber skin to wipe over the face as an instant refresher.

Sea Vegetables

This general heading includes Chinese black moss, dulse, hijiki,
kelp, kombu, mekabu, nori, plankton and wakame. In some
countries, seaweed is available as a fresh vegetable food but in
others only in its dried form from health food stores and
delicatessens. Prized by the Ancient Greeks and Romans and
the Chinese for their medicinal properties, seaweeds from non-
toxic waters provide valuable minerals including calcium,
chromium, cobalt, iron, iodine, manganese and zinc.
Unfortunately, many seas are now so polluted that these once
valuable vegetables may also be laced with cadmium, lead,
mercury, nitrates and strontium. So ask your supplier about
organic sources of seaweed for use in cooking.

Sprouted Seeds/Beans/Grains

One of the most nourishing foods ever and wonderfully good
for the skin. Try sprouting aduki beans, alfalfa, chick peas,
fenugreek seeds, lentils, millet, mung beans, pumpkin seeds,
sesame seeds or sunflower seeds. Fresh sprouts are an
abundant source of nourishment – rich in enzymes, vitamin C,
essential fatty acids, minerals, amino acids and natural sugars.

They are also one of the cheapest foods around. During germination, the concentration of nutrients increases many fold, providing the body with high-energy, low-calorie, nutrient-dense sustenance.

Preparing your own sprouts is simplicity itself. Specially designed kits are available from health food stores, but clean jam jars are just as easy to use and produce excellent results. Buy your seeds, beans and grains in small amounts and use them regularly. Check them over carefully and discard any damaged or broken ones. Rinse them thoroughly through a sieve and then fill each jar one quarter full with your chosen beans, grains or seeds, topping up with filtered water. Use either a separate jar for each variety or mix them in the same jar if you prefer. Leave to soak overnight. In the morning, pour off the water, rinse them and top up with fresh water. Repeat the procedure two or three times each day, more in hot weather. Most sprouts will be ready in three or four days – some take longer. For more detailed information on sprouting, read Leslie Kenton's wonderful book, *Raw Energy*.

Dark Green Goodness

The darker green a vegetable is, the more vitamin C, beta carotene, iron and calcium it contains – up to six times as much as a paler counterpart. Dandelion greens, dark green cabbage and lettuce, turnip greens and kale are particularly nourishing skin foods. Choose dark-leaved lettuce, too.

Herbs

Burdock Root (Arctium lappa)

Prized for its medicinal value, burdock is often partnered with dandelion or artichoke in herbal treatments. It has natural antibiotic properties, is a great liver tonic and detoxifier, an energy booster and restorative – a must in any detoxification programme – rich in iron, organic sulphur and B vitamins. Burdock has a cleansing effect upon the tissues and is recommended where mucus is a problem – such as in catarrh, sinusitis or mucus-laden stools – and for skin disorders, particularly boils, sores, poor wound healing, dry skin and eczema. Burdock root is also available for use as a fresh vegetable (try Asian greengrocery stores or Chinese delicatessens). Thin roots are the best; around one inch (two and a half centimetres) in diameter. Scrub thoroughly and slice or grate for use in stir-fries or casseroles. Burdock has a mild, earthy flavour and crunchy texture.

Dandelion (Taraxacum officinale)
For those who do not have access to fresh dandelion leaves or root, tablets and capsules are available from health food stores. Dandelion is a natural diuretic, one of the best kidney, liver and gall bladder tonics. Both the root and the leaves are excellent skin treatments, particularly where there is inflammation. Warts can be treated by applying the white sap directly to the affected areas. When treating skin disorders in my own patients, I have found dandelion and burdock to be two of the best remedies. Don't harvest dandelion leaves from the roadside – they could be contaminated with lead and other heavy metals. Always wash any collected leaves thoroughly before shredding and mixing with salads. The roots, dried, roasted or ground, make a caffeine-free coffee substitute. Most health food stores stock Dandelion 'coffee'.

Garlic (Allium sativum)
All members of the onion family, including leeks, shallots and chives, make great skin foods but garlic is in the super league

of face savers. It has natural antiseptic, antibiotic, anti-viral and anti-fungal properties, is an excellent blood tonic, natural detoxifier, antioxidant and strengthener of immune function. Garlic has been used for centuries as a wound dressing and, in several trials, has demonstrated anti-tumour activity. In the *Medical Tribune* of August 1981, a report from China showed that those who did not eat garlic were a thousand times more prone to gastric cancer than those who ate large amounts. Onions and garlic taken throughout the winter months do seem to help ward off colds and other infections. Parsley, mint and orange, lemon or grapefruit peelings help to eliminate the odour of garlic from the breath. Although still of value, fresh garlic will lose a considerable amount of its therapeutic activity once cooked, so if you are unable to tolerate raw garlic, an alternative option may be to take it as a supplement. If you use garlic tablets or capsules, always swallow them half way through a meal, rather than at the beginning or the end. This seems to help absorption, reduce any risk of indigestion and reduce the impact of any odour. Deodorized garlic does not seem to have the beneficial effects of fresh, raw or aged garlic.

Tip: If you use fresh garlic in your juicing machine, the odour may cling and taint other juices. Overcome the problem by washing the machine parts in a solution of biodegradable cleaning fluid which removes the smell of fish, onions and any other strong odours from hands, work surfaces, cooking utensils etc. (available worldwide; see Resources p.220–21).

Nettle (Urtica dioica)
The common nettle has astringent, diuretic, tonic, antirheumatic, circulatory stimulant and blood purifying properties – all beneficial in the treatment of skin problems.

Young nettle shoots are rich in vitamin C, beta carotene and mineral salts. Cook young nettle leaves like spinach, make a tisane (tea) or use as a cleansing hair rinse - good for dandruff - and face tonic.

Parsley (Petroselinum crispum)
The green curly leaves of parsley are a rich source of vitamin C, beta carotene, potassium, calcium and important trace elements boron, manganese, molybdenum and zinc. A great herbal helper for the skin, parsley is delicious in both salads and cooked dishes. The juice of fresh parsley root helps in the healing of wounds and reduces swelling. Chew fresh parsley to remove garlic odour from the breath. Mix fresh parsley sprigs with your vegetable juices.

Mint (Mentha)
Add flavour to stews, soups, salads and vegetables with chopped mint leaves. Or infuse whole leaves to make a stimulating tea (reputed to be helpful for arthritis) or to use as a refreshing mouth wash or hair rinse. Also of value as an air freshener and insect repellent.

Other Super Skin Foods

Fish
All kinds of fish are good for you but the oily ones such as mackerel, salmon, sardines and trout are particularly rich in special fatty substances called eicosapentaenoic acid and docosahexaenoic acid, essential for healthy blood, cells and skin. Fish oil, available in capsules, is showing promise as a treatment both for psoriasis and high blood pressure.

Oats

A wonderful supplier of calcium, iron, magnesium, potassium, silicon, vitamin E, B vitamins, essential fatty acids, protein and soluble dietary fibre. Apart from porridge, enjoy oat-based muesli, oat cakes and oat biscuits.

Olive Oil

One of life's most important skin savers; adding nutritious cold-pressed oils to the diet is one of the best ways to improve skin texture and moisturize from within. Rich in monounsaturated fats, now known to be extremely beneficial for healthy blood, healthy skin and for all kinds of gall bladder and liver ailments, extra virgin olive oil is guaranteed by law to be untreated by chemicals. Studies show olive oil to be helpful in balancing both blood cholesterol and blood glucose. It is highly rated as a nerve tonic, tissue strengthener and constipation remedy. Include a tablespoon per day in salad dressings or for stir-frying, even if you are following a low-fat diet. Use it externally for sunburn, minor skin eruptions and massage. Olive oil is also useful for scalp massage and as a general hair treatment. Always make sure you buy 'Extra Virgin', 'Virgin' or 'First Pressing' cold-pressed olive oil. Labels which simply say 'Pure' are not of the same high standard.

Wholegrain Rice

Brown rice provides B vitamins, calcium, magnesium, iron, zinc and gentle dietary fibre. It is easily digested and has amazing absorptive qualities for it soaks up toxins from the gut and transports them from the body. To maintain a healthy skin, detoxification and efficient elimination of wastes is vital. Brown rice is one of the best sources of skin clearing fibre. Eat plenty of other wholegrains too; there's lots of variety available, e.g. bulgur, couscous, millet, oat bran, brown pasta, quinoa and rye.

Yoghurt

One of those skin foods which is just as good for the inside of
the body as it is for the outside skin, yoghurt provides protein,
calcium, magnesium, potassium, zinc, thiamin, riboflavin and
vitamin A (although there is less vitamin A in the low-fat
varieties). Always choose yoghurts that are 'live' or 'bio' and
check for *Lactobacillus acidophilus* on the label – this is
considered most beneficial because it is a natural inhabitant of
the gut, a probiotic or 'pro-life' bacterium.

Topically, it is a nourishing face pack and also makes a useful
douche or cream application for vaginal thrush. Include a
small tub of good-quality yoghurt once or twice a week in
your diet and, if you are devoted to the low-fat kinds, check
the labels for additives, stabilizers and emulsifiers, often added
to replace the fat content. It could be healthier to eat a little
less of the unadulterated full-fat version than more additives!
Choose goat's or sheep's yoghurt if possible. For more
information on yoghurt and milk, see pp.68 and 82 and read
my book *The Food Combining Diet* (Thorsons).

Honey

This delectable sweetening has been part of man's diet since
time immemorial, firstly as wild honey and then 'cultivated' in
man-made hives; it was used by the Ancient Greeks and
Romans and recommended by Hippocrates. The subject of
wealthy anecdotal evidence, honey certainly would seem to
have some medicinal properties. Mixed with cider vinegar, it
makes a soothing cough and sore throat remedy and is helpful
for easing the pain of arthritis. A report in the *British Journal
of Surgery* (1991; 78:497–8) showed honey to be beneficial in
the treatment of superficial burns, helping wounds to heal
faster than conventional treatments. It can also be a useful

'stepping stone' for people trying to cut down on sugar. The sugar in honey is called levulose (related to the fruit sugar, fructose) and, because much of it can be absorbed into the liver without the use of insulin, puts less of a strain on the pancreas. Ordinary sugar (sucrose) needs insulin before it can be broken down and utilized. Contrary to common belief, brown sugar is no more nutritious than white. In addition, sucrose is itself nutritionally dead but has a nasty habit of using up or destroying other nutrients in the body. Good-quality honey, on the other hand, especially the darker coloured varieties, contains trace amounts of vitamins and minerals.

When choosing honey, read the labels with care. Many will use the words 'produce of more than one country' or 'blended', indicating that several honeys have been heated to mix them together. Overheating can destroy nutrients, so it's best to choose single source honey from a reputable supplier. It's worth bearing in mind that although organic honey free from pesticide sprays is likely to be a better option, the word 'organic' isn't going to mean much if the honey concerned has been heat-treated. A good guide is price: cheaper honey is nearly always blended. Some inferior brands will also lack nutrients if the bees' diet has been supplemented with sugar solution. Honey still on the comb is usually a good option. If you are in doubt about where to buy your honey, check out your local health food store.

Molasses

Apart from honey, the only sugar which is not 'pure, white and deadly' is molasses. This unrefined extraction from the sugar cane contains traces of vitamins and some important minerals – calcium, magnesium, iron, potassium, silicon – and sulphur. Another 'old' arthritis remedy, molasses is also rich in phosphoric acid, an essential cell builder which was once given to children to help improve growth and cure anaemia. A useful – and nutritious – alternative sweetener.

Nuts

These concentrated foods are often dismissed by slimmers as fattening but, although some nuts can be high in Calories, they have high energy value and are nutrient-dense. They provide valuable dietary fibre, monounsaturated and polyunsaturated oils (see p.47), worthwhile levels of protein and important minerals such as calcium, magnesium, iron and zinc. Nuts best for skin are unblanched almonds, brazils, pine nuts and macadamia nuts. Nuts are an extremely concentrated food and so should be consumed in moderation only. The oils they contain are prone to rancidity so proper storage is essential. Top-quality nuts will be unbroken (preferably still in their shells) and sold in sealed bags with a clearly marked 'use by' date. Keep all nuts in a cool dark cupboard and do not expose them to daylight or hot kitchens. If flaked nuts are required for a particular dish or recipe, break them up in a coffee grinder or processor as you need them. Peanuts are, actually, members of the pulse family and are not a recommended skin food. Unless absolutely fresh, they can carry aflatoxins (present in a fungus often invisible to the naked eye) which are potentially carcinogenic. Salted, roasted nuts are not good skin foods.

Seeds

Like nuts, seeds are a concentrated food source rich in unsaturated oils (see p.50) – excellent for the skin. Correct storage is, once again, vital so buy them in small amounts and keep them in a screw-top jar in the refrigerator. Don't choose seeds (or nuts) from serve-yourself hoppers - they will have been exposed to heat, light and air which hastens degeneration. Sunflower seeds, pumpkin seeds, linseeds, almonds, walnuts, brazils, macadamia nuts and hazelnuts all contain essential fatty acids and so make terrific skin foods. Caraway, celery, dill, fennel, fenugreek, poppy, and sesame seeds are also excellent. Avoid roasted ones; the oils they contain are likely to have been damaged.

SKIN SCOUNDRELS

The foods listed here are unlikely to help you towards healthy skin. Enjoy the occasional indulgence without feeling guilty - but avoid excesses. Too many of the 'bad guy' foods will simply undo all your good work.

- [X] All beef and beef products - apart from occasional meals of organically reared beef
- [X] All pork and pork products - including ham, pig's liver, pork pies, sausages and bacon; if you like meat, enjoy lean lamb instead
- [X] Fatty lamb (lean cuts are o.k.)
- [X] Preserved, smoked meats or smoked fish
- [X] Processed, coloured or smoked cheeses
- [X] Foods that contain long lists of E numbers and chemical-sounding names
- [X] Fatty and fried foods - especially take-aways
- [X] Refined sugar in all its forms - chocolate, sweets, ice cream, cakes, biscuits, sweet pastries, doughnuts, jam etc.
- [X] Any food which is burned, browned, seared or barbecued
- [X] Highly spiced foods
- [X] Foods with added salt and salty snacks

[X] White bread and any foods containing refined flour

[X] Wheat bran and wheat-based breakfast cereals

[X] Dried milks, dried eggs, powdered soups and coffee creamers

[X] Highly refined 'ready' meals

[X] Canned foods (exceptions: sardines and salmon, which are good sources of calcium, and fruit in natural juice, a useful emergency standby)

[X] Polyunsaturated margarines if they contain hydrogenated oils; and don't cook with polyunsaturates of any kind (see p.50)

[X] Cow's milk (see p.68)

[X] Yeast and yeasty foods

[X] Watch out for low-fat cheeses, spreads and yoghurts; emulsifiers, stabilizers, artificial flavours and colours are often used to replace the fat

[X] Excessive amounts of coffee, tea, cola, alcohol and squashes; they aggravate dehydration and increase the risk of tiny red surface veins

[X] Foods that fight i.e. proteins mixed with starches (see p.92) or any food combined with fruit

Note: Foods containing sugar or yeast are also to be avoided if you suffer from Candida Albicans, the internal yeast overgrowth which can produce a multitude of physical symptoms, notably the development or aggravation of skin problems. Following an anti-Candida diet can be very beneficial but it should be done under expert supervision, so you should consult a naturopath or dermatologist who specializes in the treatment of Candida (see also Recommended Reading).

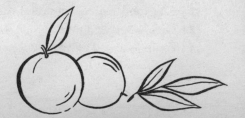

Fat Facts

I'm fat but I'm thin inside. Has it ever struck you that there's a thin man inside every fat man, just as they say there's a statue inside every block of stone.

George Orwell (Eric Arthur Blair; 1903-50), *Coming Up For Air*

Essential Fatty Acids
Ageing
Free Radical Damage
Oxygen
Antioxidants
Low-Fat Foods
Low-Fat Diets
Where to Find Healthy Fat
Sorting the Good from the Bad

UNDERSTANDING WHY CERTAIN FATS AND OILS ARE VITAL FOR HEALTHY SKIN

Whether it's on your hips or in your chips, fat has become an obsession. But the all-consuming media attention given to this villain of the diet-piece has done little to curtail the nation's corpulence or to correct its health problems.

And now a new 'illness' is creeping upon us as a result of such extreme abstinence. Fat neurosis has brought with it 'Fat Deficiency Disorders', something which I see increasingly with new patients who come to my nutrition practice.

A typical scenario is the lady who, approaching the menopause, begins to put on a bit of extra weight (often nothing more than a natural consequence of ageing and which has the benefit of providing added protection against osteoporosis, the dreaded 'brittle bone disease'). In her paranoid panic over those few additional pounds, she goes on to a 'low-fat diet' which is really a 'no-fat' diet. Common sense for good health, you might say. In moderation, certainly – reducing fat intake is believed to help lessen the risk of degenerative disease and can help to reduce weight – but taking these recommendations to extremes may cause more problems than it solves and can be particularly damaging to skin health.

Why?

DON'T TAKE LOW-FAT DIETING TOO FAR

By cutting down too far on certain types of fat, especially those unrefined liquid oils, we run the risk of becoming deficient in some very special substances called essential fatty acids. EFAs are needed by all cells in the body and are the most plentiful constituent in the membrane – or fabric – that surrounds each and every cell. Fundamental and indispensable skin nutrients, essential fatty acids help to reduce water loss from the cells, protecting the lipidic barrier between each layer of skin and preventing evaporation. They also help to build collagen and elastin fibres so, without EFAs, the plumpness and firmness of the skin is diminished, encouraging sagging, drooping and wrinkling!

EFAs play an important part in a healthy nervous system too – playing a vital role in circulation and feeding the nerve endings and sensory receptors in the skin.

Unrefined food oils are also a rich source of fatty vitamins (A, D and E) and lecithin, which acts to prevent the build-up of undesirable blocking fats, thereby reducing the risk of infection associated with oily skin, acne, spots and blemishes. Lecithin is also a very effective lubricant for dry skin.

Diets which go to fat-reducing extremes no longer contain sufficient of these vital nutrients and a list of unpleasant symptoms begin to manifest.

Most common are:

- Dry, flaky skin
- Brittle nails
- Lifeless hair
- Joint pain and stiffness
- Extreme coldness of the hands and feet
- Vaginal dryness
- Persistent viral infections
- Difficult periods
- Pre-menstrual syndrome
- Breast pain
- Loss of skin texture and premature wrinkles

These are signs that the cells may not be receiving the protection they need. More severe deficiencies could lead to inflammatory conditions such as arthritis, damage to the immune system and heart disease.

Fat is a mandatory body nutrient. Its Nemesis lies not so much in its use but in its mis-use, either inside the body or before it is consumed. Where the diet contains the wrong kinds of fats and oils in large amounts, trouble may brew. On the other hand, the right kinds in sensible quantities are absolutely, positively and definitely necessary for good health. Good skin is an impossible achievement without them and understanding the difference between good and bad fats and oils is essential in the quest for that perfect complexion.

WHAT GOES WRONG?

It's not fat which causes disease but what happens to it when it is attacked by oxygen, i.e. oxidized – like perished rubber, rusty cans and cars, or apples which go brown. Oxygen is, of course, the breath of life but, in certain circumstances, it can also act as a poison. When fats, oils and fatty foods oxidize, they 'go off' and become rancid. And fats inside the body can be attacked in a similar way, turning our natural body fats (or lipids) rancid; a process called lipid peroxidation.

FREE RADICAL FELONS

Some fats degrade more readily than others but all fats will deteriorate rapidly given 'favourable' conditions. The result is an over-production of highly active chemical compounds called free radicals, unstable substances produced as a direct result of oxygen assault.

In a healthy body, the free radicals produced as a result of normal metabolic processes are kept in check and even offer some health benefits – albeit limited. When out of control, however, free radicals behave like bad-tempered bachelors out to steal someone else's partner.

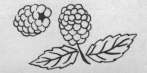

WHAT ARE THE DANGERS?

Within the body, oxygen atoms could be considered as a partnership, living together as a 'twosome'. The strength of their 'marriage' depends upon the protection supplied by the body's Argus-eyed free radical scavengers. When supplies are short, when the diet contains an overdose of undesirable fats or when the body is exposed excessively to pollution, radiation, infection, stress, smoking etc., the security screen is less effective, allowing unruly unwed free radicals to break up the relationship.

But this spouse-swapping doesn't affect just one couple. As the fanatical free radicals whizz around the body in a desperate search for a partner to join up with, they create a roller coaster effect which produces new free radicals, all out to make more mischief. The resulting havoc damages cells, causing tissues to become cross-linked (a wrinkle is the result of cross-linkage), suppressing the manufacture of new healthy cells, reducing the body's ability to fight infection and to repair damage – in other words, encouraging premature ageing and degenerative disease. Each cell in the body is governed by its own 'clock', programmed to tick for a certain length of time before running down and finally switching off. Whilst ageing and degeneration are inevitable, there are ways of shielding the system against this devastating onslaught and slowing its decline.

THE ANTIOXIDANT ARMOURY

The body has a variety of protective and scavenging mechanisms stockpiled against free radical attack. Antioxidants are the vitamins, minerals and enzymes that protect cells from oxidation (degeneration). Important antioxidant enzymes are supported by antioxidant nutrients from the diet and together they guard the cellular structure. Mother Nature also adds antioxidants (such as vitamins A, C and E, beta carotene and minerals selenium and zinc) to foods which contain susceptible fats and oils – for example, nuts, seeds and vegetables.

Trouble is, this armour is not always enough. Damaging sunlight, heat, air (oxygen, again) and radiation can speed up the oxidation process; one of the reasons why fats and oils which are reheated, overheated or left unrefrigerated in hot kitchens turn rancid so easily.

Once inside the body, degeneration can continue and will only be contained and controlled if the person's diet provides them with the antioxidant protection they need. Research shows that increasing your intake of antioxidant nutrients guards against damaging oxidation and helps to mop up free radicals, thereby slowing down the rate at which cells age and die. (For more information concerning antioxidants, vitamins and minerals read the chapter on 'Skin Nutrients', p.55.)

Evidence is emerging that these protectors may be a more significant and positive factor in the fight against ageing and disease than worrying unnecessarily over the actual levels of dietary fat.

Doctors presenting new research at the Congress of The European Society of Cardiology demonstrated that diets rich in antioxidants can protect against free radical damage and therefore reduce the risk of cell destruction and furred arteries; Drs Pauling and Rath found similar benefits during their studies with heart patients.

WHAT ABOUT LOW-FAT FOODS?

The fat in your diet provides not only a rich source of concentrated energy and nourishment but is also responsible for giving food its texture and flavour. This is why many packaged low-fat foods contain fillers, binders, emulsifiers and oodles of other additives to replace the missing fat.

In the pursuit of fat reduction, many people rely on processed products such as low-fat cheeses, low-fat yoghurts, reduced-calorie mayonnaise and fromage frais. Whilst the official advice is that these foods are perfectly healthy, I am concerned that we may be storing up further problems for the future by swapping unadulterated fat for additives and hydrogenated oils.

Kathryn Marsden's Super Skin will explain how to cut down on the potentially hazardous fats and oils and still keep your skin in great condition and your weight under control.

WHY DO WE LIKE FAT SO MUCH?

Fat fills us up and takes longer to digest than other foods; that's why, if we eat a meal with a high fat content, we feel full for longer. Hence the comfort gained from chips, crisps, cakes, pastries, doughnuts, fry-ups etc.

WHAT DO SATURATED, MONOUNSATURATED AND POLYUNSATURATED REALLY MEAN?

Fat is made up of molecules of fatty acids combined with a substance called glycerol. Each molecule is a chain-like structure of carbon atoms to which hydrogen atoms are attached. It is the shape of each structure that determines whether the fat is saturated, monounsaturated or polyunsaturated.

Sources of:		
Saturates	*Monounsaturates*	*Polyunsaturates*
Dripping	Almond	Corn (Maize)
Suet	Avocado	Fish oil
Lard	Cashew	Grapeseed
Hard margarine	Hazelnut	Linseed
Cream	Macadamia	Pumpkin seed
Cheese	Olive	Rapeseed
Milk	Pecan	Safflower
Fatty meats	Pistachio	Sesame*
Coconut		Sunflower
Butter		Walnut

* Brazil nuts, pine nuts, sesame seeds (and the oils produced from them) contain approximately equal amounts of monounsaturated and polyunsaturated oils and should therefore be treated with the respect afforded to all other polyunsaturates; in other words, avoid heating them. Whilst some authorities state that sesame oil is suitable for cooking because of its monounsaturate content, the polyunsaturates it contains are still susceptible to damage. I would therefore strongly recommend that sesame oil and seeds be kept for cold uses only.

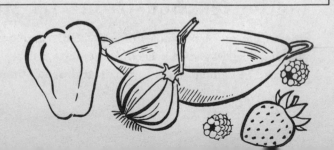

SORTING THE GOOD FROM THE NOT SO GOOD

Saturates

Saturates are those fats that tend to be solid at room temperature, like butter. Full-fat milk, cheese, cream and fatty meats are rich in saturates, the kind of fat we are usually advised to cut down on. Note, however, that there have never been any recommendations that we should give up saturated fats entirely; the body could not function properly without them. The problems lie in excess intake. Saturates can clog the arteries and slow the passage of blood and nutrients through the system. They can also overwork the lymph system (part of the body's detoxifying defences) and make it difficult for the internal 'refuse collectors' to take out the garbage. The routes of elimination become overburdened with the consequent build-up of 'junk' and the skin tries to take over some of the work. Result? Clogged pores, excess oil, pale and pasty complexion, blemishes, acne, body odour, lethargy.

Be sensible about saturates. Use them and enjoy them but in moderation only. Official U.K. guidelines recommend that saturated fats should make up only one tenth of our total calorie intake whereas dietary surveys carried out in 1992 show actual intake to be much higher, at 16 per cent.

Monounsaturates

These are found in avocado pear and olive oil and many of the nuts like macadamia and almond. New research shows that monounsaturated oils can be helpful in balancing blood glucose (good for diabetics and hypoglycaemics alike) and reducing the less desirable low-density lipoprotein (LDL cholesterol) without disturbing the levels of the beneficial HDL cholesterol or high-density lipoprotein. Check the table to find the most abundant sources of monounsaturates.

Official guidelines now recommend that these important oils should provide 12 per cent of total dietary energy. Monounsaturates also make wonderful skin, hair and nail conditioners which you'll find out about in Part Three.

Polyunsaturates

These have, for several years, been promoted as the healthy alternative to saturates and are synonymous with lowering cholesterol. Following this advice, many people dutifully dismissed their butter and jumped earnestly on to the polyunsaturated bandwagon. Unfortunately, as with so many things dietary, that counsel is now being challenged and re-examined. One of the problems is that, whilst helping to cut levels of the LDL cholesterol, polyunsaturated fatty acids (PUFAs) also reduce HDL (the cholesterol we would rather hang on to), throwing the ratio out of balance. Overdoing the polyunsaturates may not be such a healthy idea after all!

Cholesterol

In spite of what you may have been led to believe, cholesterol is *not* an illness. It is an important component of blood fat without which we would not survive. People who discover that they have elevated cholesterol levels may be panicked into thinking that a heart attack is imminent – and it is true that raised cholesterol is a heart disease risk factor. But it is one of a great many factors, including body weight, activity level, blood pressure, cigarette smoking and family history, to name a few.

If you have a high total cholesterol reading but a correspondingly high HDL to LDL ratio, some experts believe you are not at risk; but most doctors' surgeries and hospitals carry out initial tests by measuring *total* cholesterol only.

If you cut down too far on cholesterol-containing foods, your body will manufacture extra cholesterol internally to make up the shortfall. And new evidence of the incidence of heart attacks among women suggests that you may be more at risk if your cholesterol falls too far.

Polyunsaturates Fall Into Two Groups

Real polyunsaturates are not spreading fats but oils found mainly in vegetables, nuts, seeds and oily fish. Corn, rapeseed, safflower and sunflower are the most familiar of the polyunsaturated oils found on our grocery or supermarket shelves. Once extracted from their host plant, real polys remain naturally liquid at room temperature. If undamaged by processing and carefully stored, they are rich in essential fatty acids and of great value to the diet. The body cannot produce its own polyunsaturated fatty acids and it is imperative that these vital nutrients are provided from the food we eat.

But polyunsaturates should not form the bulk of our fat intake. Department of Health recommendations suggest only 6 per cent of our total daily calorie intake should come from a combination of polyunsaturated plant and fish oils.

To Get The Most From Your Polys, Follow These Simple Rules

- Choose the best quality you can find. Price is a reliable guide since the more expensive oils are nearly always more nutritious. Look for the words 'cold pressed' on the label, indicating that the oil has not been damaged by over-processing or the use of solvents.

- Buy in small quantities and use up well within the recommended date.
- Never, never, never use polyunsaturates of any kind for anything that requires heating or cooking. The increase in temperature encourages the formation of lipid peroxides, dangerous and potentially carcinogenic substances. So, keep them for salad dressings and mayonnaise only. Chips cooked in polyunsaturated oil are not healthier than those cooked in animal fat!
- Don't leave oils standing in a hot kitchen or in daylight, two of the speediest ways to turn them rancid. Store them in a cool, dark cupboard or, better still, in the refrigerator. I believe that manufacturers should be encouraged to use dark glass bottles instead of clear glass or plastic.
- Always replace the cap securely.

The health-giving structure of polyunsaturates is altered, detrimentally, if they are over-processed, heated, subjected to light, air, radiation or environmental pollution, stripped of their natural antioxidant protectors such as vitamin E - or hydrogenated.

Hydrogenation
Hydrogenation is a manufacturing process which takes the liquid polyunsaturated oil and alters its chemical structure to make it into a solid - the reason why your sunflower margarine doesn't run off the side of the kitchen worktop! Check the label for the words 'made from hydrogenated vegetable oils'. Whilst most of these products will proclaim that they are 'rich

in polyunsaturates' and 'low in saturates', the hydrogenation process actually alters some of the polys into saturates as well as damaging the essential fatty acids. Another generally unpublicized fact is that a great many polyunsaturated spreads contain the same amount of fat as saturates!

The manufacturers of hydrogenated spreads often see these kinds of explanations as an attack on their products. Needless to say, they are anxious to prove to the public that their 'margarines' are safe and that there is no evidence to suggest that long-term use is a problem. However, the 1991 Committee on Medical Aspects of Food Policy has accepted that the existing evidence available on polyunsaturated fatty acids justifies a cautious approach.

The number of studies questioning the value of this manufacturing process are gathering. Since there is unlikely to be smoke without fire, it may be foolhardy to treat hydrogenation as 'a safe process until proven otherwise'. My nutritionist's instincts incline me to the more guarded approach that we should avoid them until their benefits/hazards have been evaluated objectively and independently by researchers who can declare no vested interests in the food industry or its sales.

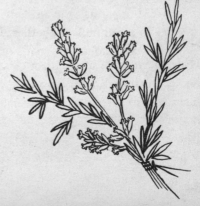

HERE'S HOW TO CUT FAT INTAKE BUT STILL ENJOY REAL FOOD!

- Eat more fresh fish and free-range poultry.
- Cut down on red meat, particularly beefburgers, sausages, bacon, pork pies and pasties.
- Be sensible about sticky buns, cakes, biscuits, chocolate, ice cream and crisps. Enjoy them only as very occasional treats.
- Stir-fry, grill, poach, bake or casserole your food. Never deep fry anything.
- Use extra virgin olive oil (instead of polyunsaturates) for cooking. It's more stable when heated and less prone to rancidity (although the careful storage guidelines still apply).
- For spreading, avoid margarines that are made with hydrogenated vegetable oils (check the labels) and use either small amounts of butter or non-hydrogenated spreads – available from health food stores.
- Avoid low-fat foods of the processed variety, especially if they contain lots of artificial additives and chemical-sounding names.
- Where you are torn between the low-fat soft cheese or low-fat yogurt and the full-fat alternatives, choose the latter but eat half the amount.
- Try to avoid milk altogether. If you find this difficult, use small amounts of goat's or sheep's milk and dilute with 25 per cent water – or go for semi-skimmed milk and restrict intake to one quarter pint daily.

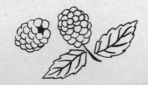

Skin Nutrients

A good kitchen is a good Apothicaries shop.

William Bullein (d.1576), *The Bulwark Against All Sickness*

> Antioxidants
> Vitamins
> Minerals
> Essential Fatty Acids
> Royal Jelly
> Probiotics
> Antibiotics
> Deficiency Signs and Symptoms
> Supplement Safety

A keen gardener may spend hours digging, weeding and hoeing the beds and borders in order to produce a beautifully manicured appearance. But if the nutrients in the soil are lacking or are not replaced, then the plants growing there will eventually suffer. Similarly, the skin will deteriorate if the body is poorly nourished and lacking in the vitamins, minerals, amino-acids, enzymes and hormones that all act synergistically to renew healthy cells.

It can be interesting – and helpful – to understand the action of antioxidants and some of the other major nutrients involved in skin function and to know which foods supply the richest sources.

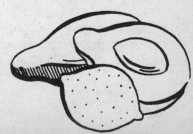

VITAMINS

Vitamin A

Vitamin A is an essential skin nutrient and is found in the diet in two basic forms:

1. Beta Carotene is an important anti-ageing, antioxidant nutrient found in carotenoid foods; for example, cantaloup melons, apricots, pumpkins, carrots, swedes, turnips, parsley, endive, squash, sweet potatoes, plankton and green leafy vegetables. In fact, most orange, yellow and dark green produce contains beta carotene. It is also a precursor of vitamin A; in other words, in ideal conditions the body will convert beta carotene into vitamin A in the small intestine and liver.

2. Retinol is the vitamin A available from animal foods such as lamb's liver, oily fish, fish oil supplements, eggs and cheese. An overdose of vitamin A from diet would be difficult to achieve but, since excesses of this vitamin can be toxic, it is wise to be cautious. (Retinol is not to be confused, however, with the vitamin A-based drug Retin A – see p.137.) Where a deficiency is suspected or additional amounts required, ask for professional guidance on supplementation, especially if you are pregnant or planning a baby. However, do bear in mind that deficiencies are as dangerous as excesses. Vitamin A is essential for a healthy pregnancy and studies show its importance in the prevention and treatment of dangerous childhood illnesses such as measles.

A lack of vitamin A damages cell membranes. New cells die off before they have a chance to reach the surface, blocking the pores and preventing lubrication of the skin.

Both kinds of vitamin A are widely available from food and yet the symptoms of deficiency are extremely common. You could be short of vitamin A if you suffer with:

Dry, rough and scaly skin	Spots, boils and pimples
Whiteheads, blackheads	Frequent, recurring skin infections
Throat infections	Mouth ulcers
Cystitis	Thrush
Dandruff	Dry hair
Night blindness	Sore, burning, itchy eyes
Inflamed eyelids	Flaking, peeling nails

Vitamin A enhances the activity of essential fatty acids, particularly gamma linolenic acid (GLA); it works closely with zinc to support immune function and helps to transport other life-sustaining nutrients to the cells. Many scientific researches have shown vitamin A and beta carotene to be linked to reduced cancer risk and long-term studies continue with promising results. For more information, Caroline Wheater's book *Beta Carotene* (Thorsons) makes useful reading.

The B Complex Group of Vitamins
Includes:
Thiamin (B_1)
Riboflavin (B_2)
Nicotinic Acid – sometimes also called Niacin (B_3)
Pantothenic Acid (B_5)
Pyridoxine (B_6)

Folic Acid (B_9)
Cobalamin (B_{12})
Biotin (also known as vitamin H)

Choline and Inositol are also members of the B group but are not strictly vitamins since they can be manufactured within the body. Para-aminobenzoic acid (PABA) is also part of this group but should be regarded as a B factor, not a true vitamin.

In my experience with patients, the B vitamins are usually found lacking when there are skin problems. They are needed for the repair and rebuilding of tissue, for feeding the endocrine and nervous systems and for energy production.

Vitamin B deficiency symptoms include:

Pale skin	Generally poor skin condition
Cracks, splits or sores around the nose and mouth	Sore, itchy eyes
Pre-menstrual syndrome	Irregular, heavy or painful periods
Extreme fatigue	Lack of energy
Twitchy, restless limbs	Tingling or 'burning' in the legs or arms
Difficulty with memory	A tendency to drop or bump into things
Nervous disorders	Panic attacks

B vitamins turn up in a wide variety of foodstuffs. The best natural sources are seeds, nuts, wholegrains, lamb's liver, dark green vegetables and legumes.

If you are plagued by skin problems, try taking extra B vitamins for three months. Most good-quality multi formulas or B complexes will provide 25 – 50mg of each B vitamin.

Vitamin C

Another super antioxidant nutrient, vital for fighting infection, for wound healing and the formation of collagen, often referred to as the cement that holds the skin together. Collagen degeneration can be linked to a lack of vitamin C and when the elasticity of collagen collapses, skin sags and ages very quickly. Vitamin C has hundreds of other biochemical tasks too. It reduces the risk of arterial damage and cardiovascular disease, balances blood cholesterol, protects against stress, reduces allergic reactions and is needed for energy production.

Common signs of vitamin C deficiency are:

Frequent colds/infections	Easy bruising
Bleeding gums	Cystitis
Constipation	Haemorrhoids (piles)
Broken capillaries	Cuts that won't heal
Clogged arteries	High cholesterol

'Expensive urine' is the oft-touted argument aired by those who believe we should be able to obtain all our vital nutrients from diet alone. Vitamin C is water soluble; the body needs a daily supply because water-soluble nutrients are not stored by the system. Some doctors are convinced that it is a waste of time taking more vitamin C than the official Recommended Daily Amount (now called the RNI or Reference Nutrient Intake) because excesses will be wasted via the urine.

However, more and more studies demonstrate that, for the majority of the population, extra vitamin C can be beneficial. Human beings are one of the few animal species no longer able to manufacture their own vitamin C. Most people need levels far above the officially recommended amount before any vitamin C shows up in the urine. In addition, vitamin C protects the bowel, bladder and kidneys – so even that which does pass through is of benefit. Diarrhoea is sometimes listed as a detrimental 'side effect' of vitamin C supplementation. In fact, one of the clearest naturopathic indicators of vitamin C requirement for any individual is the level they are able to tolerate before experiencing a loose bowel. In other words, if a patient increases his daily dose of vitamin C to, say, 5 grams before he has diarrhoea, then 4 grams per day is likely to be his natural requirement.

If you are a worrier, suffer from stress and anxiety, work in a polluted atmosphere, are surrounded by electrical and electronic equipment or travel regularly in heavy traffic, try supplementing your diet with one or two grams daily of vitamin C complex. Choose a product that also contains Bioflavonoids, natural partners to vitamin C and essential for healthy, strong blood vessels (see below, p.62).

Avoid the kind of vitamin C that effervesces in water. Much of its usefulness is lost during the 'fizzing' action. And steer clear of products that are labelled 'ascorbic acid' – they can be too acidic and often upset the digestion. If only the smallest doses of vitamin C cause stomach pain and/or diarrhoea, this – in my experience – is usually due to a poor-quality ascorbic acid product which has irritated the gut lining. Buffered or low-acid formulas (labels include the word 'ascorbate') are more gentle and beneficial.

Make sure your diet contains lots of vitamin C-rich foods such as blackcurrants, acerola cherries, kiwi fruits (there is twice as much vitamin C in a single kiwi fruit as in a large orange), apricots, grapefruit, kumquats, guava, papaya, green leafy vegetables and saladings, kohlrabi, turnip tops, parsley, green and red peppers and jacket potatoes. Most fruits and vegetables contain some vitamin C so aim for two or three pieces of fruit, a good helping of fresh vegetables and a salad every day.

Note: There is some concern that additional vitamin C may make oestrogen more active so, if you are taking the contraceptive pill, swallow your vitamin C at a different time of day.

Vitamin C Cream

Vitamin C is well known for its role in skin health, its ability to give antioxidant protection, reduce inflammation and speed healing. Apart from food sources, it can be taken as powders, tablets or capsules or administered by injection.

When skin is grazed, burned or cut, the damaged area can be sealed over and protected on the surface against bacterial invasion and further harm, but the actual healing takes place from inside the body. All skin ages from the inside out as the body's mechanisms for replacing cells begins to diminish. And the ageing process is aggravated from the outside too, ravaged by pollution, sun exposure and other external damage.

Surface application of cosmetics helps to lubricate and protect the outer layers of skin but the race is still on to find an anti-ageing cream which will slow or stop those dreaded wrinkles. Some substances such as aloe vera (whose high levels of zinc make it a natural astringent) and vitamin E are very useful for topical application and can help to enhance internal repair, but very few nutrients are able to penetrate and heal damaged skin from the outside in – which is why the majority of the body's nourishment must be fed via the mouth and digestive system.

Scientists working for the Australian government have achieved a world first by producing a vitamin C cream able to penetrate the skin and saturate the underlying tissue within 30 minutes of topical application. In extensive and repeated studies, as little as 2 grams of the cream was able to raise the deep tissue concentrations of the nutrient by 10,000 per cent! After the vitamin C has been completely diffused, it then moves on to nourish the circulation.

Produced by a special patented process, the cream (called Derma-C) is entirely additive-free, containing only vitamin C and glycerate. During tests, wide-ranging benefits were discovered: Derma-C is known to support the healing process by strengthening the collagen in capillaries, joints and tendons, reducing inflammation and acting as a local antioxidant to scavenge for free radicals. It has a rapid soothing effect on traumatized tissue and helps to reduce minor pain in the joints. Clinical experience also shows it to be beneficial in the treatment of scalds, grazing, bruises, skin rashes and muscle pain. It appears to reduce the inflammation and discomfort associated with arthritic joints and which follows knee joint surgery. (For more information, see Resources.)

Bioflavonoids
Also known as citrus salts or flavones. Once thought to be a vitamin and so still sometimes referred to as the vitamin P complex.

Bioflavonoids are found with vitamin C in plant foods and are the major source of their red and blue pigments. (The carotenes supply the majority of orange, dark green and yellow colour.) Best known sources of bioflavonoids are fresh apricots, beetroot, bilberries, blackcurrants, broccoli, buckwheat, cantaloup melon, cherries, papaya, and the pith and skin of citrus fruits (particularly lemons).

When choosing bioflavonoid supplements, once again price is a good guide to quality. For example, products containing potent and active flavonoids – such as gingko biloba and/or bilberry – are likely to be more expensive (but more effective) than cheaper brands sourced from citrus fruits. (See Resources.)

If you suffer with any of the following symptoms, then increase the beneficial food sources listed above and consider taking a bioflavonoid supplement for three to four months:

Broken veins	Easy bruising
Haemorrhoids (piles)	Varicose veins/ulcers
Unexplained nosebleeds	Bleeding gums

Bioflavonoids have been found to be beneficial in the treatment of fluid retention, varicose veins, heavy menstrual bleeding, allergies, haemorrhage, diabetic retinopathy and high blood pressure. Anecdotal evidence suggests they may also be useful in treating fatigue. Their outstanding anti-inflammatory and antioxidant properties make them superlative skin nutrients, helping to maintain the integrity of blood vessels and capillaries, reducing pain, bruising and bleeding. They protect against free radical attack, shield vitamin C from damage and enhance its favourable effects. Some kinds of bioflavonoids are able to adhere themselves to collagen fibres to offer additional defence and restore flexibility and resilience.

Collagen, the intercellular cement, is a protein substance which, with elastin, gives skin its elasticity, strength and support. Healthy collagen cannot be produced or repaired without vitamin C or bioflavonoids. Some bioflavonoid substances are also believed to provide both external and internal sunscreen protection.

It's interesting to note that, half a century ago, bioflavonoids were produced and sold by leading pharmaceutical companies to treat haemorrhage and capillary fragility. Despite being particularly effective and very safe, this practice ceased when it was discovered that these natural substances could not be patented. (For 'not patentable', read 'not profitable'!)

Vitamin D

It has long been known that vitamin D is an essential requirement for strong bones and teeth but new research suggests that it may also play a part in improving bone density *after* the age at which bone growth is said to be completed: usually between the ages of thirty and forty. Vitamin D is found in foods such as oily fish and eggs and is also produced by the action of daylight on the skin; one of the reasons why it is so important to spend time out of doors even on overcast days.

In one study, post-menopausal women who were given small amounts of additional vitamin D (equivalent to only one half hour's sunlight exposure per day) showed a significant increase in bone strength. In another, wintertime bone loss was reduced and bone density improved in women who took vitamin D. In a third, increases in bone mineralization were demonstrated in subjects who took additional calcium in an easily assimilated form. Without vitamin D, calcium cannot be properly utilized within the body. You may see small amounts of vitamin D included in good-quality multivitamin preparations. However, separate supplements of vitamin D are not widely available and, because of the risk of overdosing, should only ever be used under practitioner supervision.

Vitamin E

Now scientifically proven in the prevention and treatment of heart disease and circulatory disorders, vitamin E is also *the* vitamin for reducing scarring following accident or surgery. It can even reduce the prominence of old scars if applied regularly and has been used to help burn victims. Vitamin E is known to prolong cell life, improve skin quality, prevent blood clotting and hasten wound healing.

All kinds of skin conditions from the very dry to the very oily, including eczema, acne, psoriasis, sunburn, scalds and stretch marks, can be helped by topical applications of vitamin E. I have found that the best way to apply vitamin E is to pierce a capsule with a sterilized needle and massage it gently into the skin with clean fingers. Although wheatgerm oil is often suggested as a rich source of vitamin E for this purpose, it has a very short shelf life and is prone to rapid rancidity once opened. It may even have become rancid at the point of processing and bottling.

Extra vitamin E can be helpful where there is:

Dry skin	Scarring
Heart disease	High blood pressure
Hormonal imbalance	Easy bruising
Stress	Poor circulation

Vitamin E protects unsaturated fatty acids and other fat-soluble nutrients from attack by oxygen. When fats and oils are refined – or their chemical structure altered – vitamin E is destroyed, so if your diet is high in processed foods and hydrogenated spreads, you could benefit from taking additional vitamin E as a supplement. But avoid large doses, which are unnecessary and could be dangerous. A daily amount of 100iu to 400iu (as part of a multi-complex formula) will give good antioxidant protection.

Richest food sources are cold-pressed oils, all kinds of seeds, nuts (particularly almonds), wholegrains (especially brown rice), eggs, fruits, asparagus, sprouted grains and green vegetables. Avoid wheatgerm flakes, however, which harbour the same storage and rancidity problems as wheatgerm oil.

MINERALS

Calcium

Calcium has many roles in the body apart from being the major constituent in our teeth and bones. Without it, nerves would not function, skin and muscles would lack tone and strength, blood vessels would weaken and skin would not heal.

Calcium is also an important factor in the metabolism of essential fatty acids and - with vitamin C - in the manufacture of collagen, and it works closely with other nutrients to maintain healthy skin.

Calcium deficiency can lead to:

Bone pain	Easily broken bones
Slow healing and mending of fractures	Panic attacks
Muscle spasms and twitching, particularly of the limbs	
Insomnia	Depression

As with all minerals, absorption of calcium can be hampered by many factors:

[X] Too many saturated fats in the diet can form insoluble soaps with calcium, so keep saturates to sensible limits

[X] Rhubarb; apart from being uncomfortably acidic, it contains oxalates which bind to calcium and prevent its absorption

[X] The phytates in unrefined grains do much the same thing, so steer clear of coarse wheat bran - the sawdust sprinkled over breakfast cereals

[X] Calcium doesn't like diets that contain too much phosphorus (found in red meat, carbonated drinks, junk food)

[X] Stomach acid is needed to dissolve calcium prior to absorption. If you experience persistent indigestion immediately after meals, you could be suffering from an under-acid stomach (hypochlorhydria), often mistaken for over-acidity

☒ Excess use of aluminium-based antacids can prevent calcium absorption

☒ Vitamin D (converted by the skin from daylight) is absolutely essential if calcium is to be properly utilized. Try to spend some time outdoors every day if possible

☒ Diets rich in animal protein cause calcium to be excreted in excess by the kidneys

☒ Lactose intolerance – the inability to digest milk sugar – will prevent absorption of calcium from milk. But there are plenty of other calcium-rich foods to choose from (see below)

☒ Lack of magnesium – this mineral must be present for calcium to be properly assimilated so it's important to include magnesium containing nuts, wholegrains, fresh fruit and vegetables in the diet

Milk is generally put forward as the best supplier of calcium but it is not well digested by everyone. Cow's milk is an infamous allergen, well known for causing gastric upset, catarrh and a range of other symptoms and is not recommended as a good (internal) food for skin. (However, milk can be useful as a topical cleanser and moisturizer.)

There are lots of other beneficial sources of calcium to choose from: canned fish (especially sardines and salmon), cheese, nuts, seeds, pulses, root vegetables, green vegetables, oatmeal, brown rice, eggs and fresh fish are just a few, although this mineral is abundant in a wide range of foods.

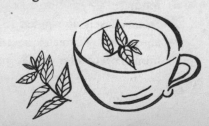

Chromium

It has been said that the total amount of chromium required by one human being for a whole lifetime would fill only an egg cup - and yet, because of intensive farming, crop spraying, food processing and high-sugar diets, this trace mineral is one of the most commonly deficient.

Essential for controlling blood glucose levels and for balancing blood fats and cholesterol, you could be short of chromium if you have:

Excessive thirst	Poor co-ordination
Excessive sweating – particularly night sweats	Dizziness or poor concentration after more than three hours without eating
Need for frequent meals	Waking hungry during the night
High blood fats and/or high cholesterol	Drowsiness during the day
Chronic fatigue or sudden unexplained exhaustion	
Hypoglycaemia	Family history of diabetes

Best food sources of chromium are lamb's liver, blackstrap molasses, cheese, seafood, wholegrains, egg yolk, raw beetroot, plankton, spirulina and asparagus.

By reducing the risk of hypoglycaemia and diabetes, good chromium levels also guard, indirectly, against nervous system damage such as diabetic neuropathy. It can also reduce elevated triglycerides and high cholesterol.

Iron

Population studies carried out around the world would suggest that iron deficiency is extremely common. For example, an Australian dietary survey published in 1988 showed 45 per cent of women to be low in iron - and also in calcium, zinc, magnesium and vitamins A, C and B$_6$. A similar U.K. investigation of 800 people indicated that 60 per cent of women had iron intakes below the RDA.

In food, iron exists in two different forms: organic haem iron is abundant in meat foods, from which it is generally well absorbed. Inorganic non-haem iron is the kind found in vegetables, fruits and nuts and must be altered chemically by the body before it can be used. This is why vegetarians are advised to eat iron-rich vegetables with those containing vitamin C, since the vitamin helps to carry the iron across the intestinal wall into the bloodstream. Malic acid, found in plums, apples and pumpkin, and the citric acid in citrus fruits, also enhance the absorption of 'veggie' iron.

Interestingly, however, iron deficiency appears to be rare in vegans and vegetarians but widespread among the population as a whole, as confirmed by a 1985 *British Medical Journal* report by Barber, Bull and Buss which stated that young meat-eating women were consuming iron at 25 per cent below the recommended daily amounts.

Iron is an essential trace mineral needed to make haemoglobin - the red pigment in blood cells - and myoglobin, another iron-containing pigment which carries and stores oxygen in muscle tissue. Iron is also an important constituent in a number of enzymes and is vital for healthy growth and mental development. If iron stores are low the body will try to compensate by absorbing more from food, but when reserves fall too far the result is iron-deficiency anaemia.

Suspect iron deficiency if you notice:

Paler than usual skin	Pale nails
Persistent, abnormal fatigue	Brittle nails
Lack of red colour inside	
the lower eyelid	Dry hair
Difficult breathing	Palpitations
Loss of appetite	Indigestion
Continual, unexplained	
headaches with dizziness	
and/or visual disturbance	

Vitamin B_{12} is essential for the absorption of iron and may be lacking if you are experiencing digestive discomfort, have a bright red tongue or suffer with nervous disorders, tingling in the fingers and toes or poor co-ordination. Iron absorption may also be inhibited where there is insufficient vitamin C, vitamin A, folic acid or copper or an excess of zinc. Problems of deficiency may be further aggravated by aspirin-based drugs, lack of stomach acid, too much cereal fibre in the diet or too many cups of tea or canned fizzy drinks.

Anyone concerned that they are anaemic or unable to consume enough iron should ask their doctor for a blood test before launching into self-prescribed iron tablets. Most types of iron supplement are notoriously poorly absorbed and well known for their gut irritant and constipating talents – and overdosing on iron could be dangerous. If you have iron supplements in the house, keep them right away from youngsters. As little as 3mg could kill a small child.

Note: One of the most easily assimilated and gentle forms of iron supplement for adults is called Iron Ethanol Amine Phosphate (Iron EAP2); especially helpful for those people who cannot tolerate Ferrous sulphate (see Resources).

Best sources of iron from food are lamb's liver, sardines, wholegrains, pulses, nuts, seeds, dried fruit, parsley, watercress, beetroot, broccoli, cabbage, celery, endive, sweet potato, tomatoes, turnip, apples, bananas, eggs and blackstrap molasses.

Magnesium
Not only is magnesium a vital partner to calcium, it also assists the B vitamins and essential fatty acids so fundamental for healthy skin. It works to repair and maintain cells and tissues, balance hormones and support the nervous system.

If you are short of magnesium, you might notice symptoms such as:

Twitchy muscles	Restless limbs
Muscle weakness	Muscle spasm
Period problems	Pre-menstrual syndrome
Palpitations	Breathlessness
Insomnia	Depression or anxiety
Constipation	Dizziness
Sweating	Poor co-ordination
Unexplained fatigue	Cramp

Good food sources of magnesium are nuts – particularly cashews, almonds and brazils – sesame seeds, haricot beans, brown rice, wholegrain flour, seafoods, bananas, dark green vegetables, phytoplankton, sprouted seeds and dried fruit. Many varieties of vegetables contain small but valuable amounts of this important skin mineral.

Selenium

A trace element, needed only in tiny quantities, selenium forms a vital part of the antioxidant enzyme glutathione peroxidase. The functions of selenium include the maintenance of healthy skin and hair, providing protection against free radical activity and pollution as well as supporting immune function. Epidemiological evidence shows that selenium is frequently deficient in patients with cancer, rheumatoid arthritis and heart disease. It works synergistically with vitamins C and E, both important antioxidant skin protectors and also plays an important anti-inflammatory role in the body.

Selenium deficiency signs include:

Hair, skin and nail
problems
Dry, flaking skin   Poor wound healing
Brittle, flaking nails   Bleeding nails
Stiff and painful joints   Poor resistance to infection
High blood pressure   Angina

You should be able to find selenium in fish and shellfish, wholegrains – particularly brown rice, eggs, milk, fruits and vegetables. Unfortunately, soil deficiency of this mineral is common.

Zinc

The benefits that zinc bestows to the skin should not be underestimated. Some experts believe zinc deficiency to be epidemic - and my own experience with patients would certainly suggest that low zinc levels are extremely common, particularly where skin problems are concerned.

Without zinc, vitamin A cannot be properly utilized. Zinc is vital for growth and repair, for wound healing, balancing insulin production and for helping other hormones.

Symptoms of zinc deficiency include:

Excessively dry or excessively oily skin	Acne
Slow wound healing	Persisting infections
Poor hair quality	Loss of taste or smell
White marks on the fingernails	
Blood sugar disorders	Poor appetite
Poor digestion (may be connected to low levels of stomach acid)	Infertility

---

Good dietary sources include fish, meat, cheese, milk, vegetables, nuts, seeds, grains, plankton and kelp. Even where the diet is well supplied, however, absorption can be poor because zinc competes with other minerals - such as calcium - for transport across the gut wall. Food additives can affect, adversely, the absorption of zinc as can too much of the wrong kind of dietary fibre. For this reason, it is probably wise to avoid wheat bran and wheat-based cereals, choosing wholegrain rye, rice, oats, buckwheat and millet instead.

If an additional zinc supplement becomes necessary, it is best taken first thing in the morning or last thing at night away from other nutrients. Do not supplement for long periods of time without a break or without the support of a varied and nourishing diet as this could result in multiple imbalances of other nutrients.

ESSENTIAL FATTY ACIDS

Essential fatty acids (EFAs) are just that – essential – because they must be provided in the diet and cannot be produced by the body. EFAs have many vital functions within the system. They are active in the structure of cell membranes; they increase oxygen uptake and are an important component in energy production. The balance of hormones within the body is detrimentally affected by a deficiency or malfunction of fatty acids; so is muscle tone.

There are plenty of different sources of essential fatty acids in foods, for example, fish (which contains alpha-linolenic acid or ALA), vegetables, pulses, seeds and nuts (rich in linoleic acid or LA). However, despite this dietary abundance, EFA deficiency remains extremely common.

To be of any use to the body, the fatty acids from the food have to be converted before they can be used: alpha-linolenic acid to the almost unpronounceable eicosapentanoic and docosahexanoic acids (EPA and DHA for short) and the linoleic acid to gamma-linolenic acid (GLA) and di-homo gamma-linolenic acid (DGLA). Complicated stuff! All these EFAs are required to produce very important hormone-like substances called prostaglandins, biological 'communicators' which are a fundamental part of all body processes.

As explained in the chapter 'Fat Facts', the conversion process is easily thwarted – by stress, pollution, toxicity, infections, deficiencies of other nutrients and a poor-quality or unbalanced diet.

Scientific studies have shown that supplementing with GLA and fish oils can overcome the blocked metabolic pathway and give considerable relief to a range of diseases commonly associated with a lack of EFAs, for example:

Eczema	Psoriasis
Mastalgia	Pre-menstrual syndrome
Heart and circulatory disorders	
Viral infections	Post-viral fatigue
Multiple Sclerosis	Diabetes

GLA has also been shown to be of benefit in maintaining skin moisture and increasing its smoothness.

When choosing essential fatty acids as a supplement, it is important to look for high-quality products. Safe and effective ones will not be cheap so, as a *very* general rule, buy the most expensive you can afford. If you choose evening primrose oil, the recommended dose is 4–6 capsules of 500mg each daily. When buying dedicated GLA complexes, you may need to take less because specific GLA products are often more concentrated.

It is best to avoid essential fatty acids sold in liquid form. Many have been subjected to oxygen contamination during the bottling process and will, therefore, have no beneficial effect on the body. Even those that are produced under stringent conditions will have a very short shelf life.

CO-ENZYME Q10

When it comes to the really big guns of the *Antioxidant Armoury* (see p. 45), one particularly important defender is a vitamin-like substance called Co-enzyme Q10 – also known as Ubiquinone or Q10 for short. Scientists now believe that deficiency of Q10 may be widespread and that, although the nutrient is found in limited amounts in the diet, there may not be enough to provide long-term health protection. Q10 is known to have a positive influence on the immune system and on the ageing process!

Now available as a supplement, the recommended daily dose is 30mg to 90mg. Best taken in capsule form together with a multivitamin/mineral or antioxidant complex that contains vitamins A, C, E, B_5, B_6, manganese, magnesium, selenium and zinc. Anyone requiring further information on the research into and uses of Q10 should contact Pharma Nord UK (see Resources for details). For details of stockists of Q10 and antioxidant supplements, see Resources on p. 218.

PROBIOTICS

From the Greek *bios* ('life'); 'pro-biotic' or 'pro-bios' means 'pro-life'.

When looking at vital body nutrients, probiotics are an often-overlooked factor. Since they play such an important role in maintaining the health of the skin, have much needed antioxidant capabilities and are a powerful force in restoring the status quo after antibiotics, it can help to understand their basic functions.

'Antibiotic' means 'an anti-bacterial agent'; 'a substance capable of destroying or injuring living organisms especially bacteria'. Anti-bios or antibiotic could therefore be translated as 'anti-life'. Whilst acknowledging the value of these drugs as a first-line treatment in many life-endangering situations, they continue to be mis-prescribed and over-used. Ultimately, I believe, indiscriminate use may play a significant part in destroying or injuring the very 'living organisms' they were designed to save – us! It seems that every success holds within itself the seeds of its own destruction.

Teenagers Suffer

For example, long-term use of tetracyclines, one of the favoured suppressive treatments for teenage acne, has done nothing to eradicate the cause of this depressing condition.

At a time in their lives when looking their best becomes all-important, anxious adolescents are faced not just with pimples but side effects such as bowel disorders, thrush, compromised immunity and a range of other difficulties caused, exclusively, by their medication. Recommending, as a first resort, the use of antibiotics to people with acne and other skin disorders is, in my view, totally irresponsible. The apparent short-term gain can turn all too horribly into a serious health problem: the over-use of antibiotics may be responsible, some experts believe, for the increased incidence of some immune-related illnesses. Probiotics, on the other hand, have been shown to be especially helpful in the treatment of acne and other skin conditions (see chapter entitled 'Acne Attack').

Antibiotics in Food

Apart from doctors' prescriptions, antibiotics are regularly injected into farm animals or added to their feed to prevent the spread of infection in cramped, intensive farming units. Even though there is an official waiting period between antibiotic administration and slaughter, it is inevitable that residues of these drugs find their way into the food chain to be ingested later by human beings or other animals. For this reason, it is wise to avoid battery-raised poultry and battery eggs and intensively reared beef and pork. Wherever possible, go for organic, free-range sources.

Superbugs

Non-selective and careless employment of antibiotics has brought with it superbugs, bacteria which are now resistant to many of the prescription medicines currently available.

But instead of looking at more natural ways to overcome these problems, the powerful pharmaceutical companies see irresistible opportunities to make matters worse, spending millions each day researching and developing even more potent pills. It is estimated that, every year, they mail the average G.P. his own weight in advertising material and it is alleged that they spend thousands per doctor on 'inducements' to buy their products. Profits continue to rise – but at what cost?

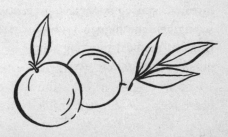

Many drugs are dangerous and toxic, not even effective in curing the condition for which they were prescribed. A quick glance at any doctor's drug 'bible' will reveal that most prescribed medicines produce side effects which, in many cases, require the need for further drugs to overcome them.

It is said that around ten per cent of hospital beds in the U.K. are occupied by patients who were prescribed the wrong medication. In the United States, over one million people a year end up in hospital as a result of negative reactions to drugs. (These figures do not include deliberate overdoses, addiction to hard drugs or suicides.)

It isn't my intention to malign the medics; merely to point out that all is not as rosy as it might appear in conventional medicine country. No-one would deny the amazing advances in modern medical practice; life-saving heart operations, limb-saving microsurgery, the paramedic expertise of the emergency services or the fact that, because of insulin, diabetes is no longer a killer illness. But as Bernie Siegel so cannily reminds us, 'M.D.' does not stand for 'Medical Deity'. It might be just as well for us to remember that the word 'doctor' also means to 'botch', 'cobble', 'patch up', 'disguise', 'falsify' and 'tamper with'.

I cannot help feeling that the cache of scientific expertise and cash currently devoted to new drug research might be better invested in protection and prevention – studying products that strengthen the human immune system to withstand attack. Current medical thinking seems to favour waiting for illness to attack before taking action.

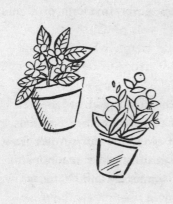
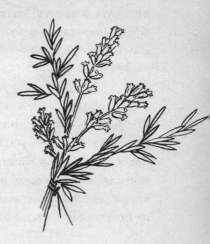

Which Bugs Are Which?

The gastrointestinal tract is home to a wide variety of bacteria which can be split into two main categories: the beneficial *Bifido* bacteria and *acidophilus* (*lactobacilli*; i.e. they produce lactic acid), and the not-so-friendly Bacteroides micro-organisms. The *Bifido* and *lactobacillus acidophilus* bacteria have an important role to play in the synthesis of some important vitamins and encourage the absorption of certain minerals; they also have natural antibiotic, antioxidant and anti-tumour tendencies. Where health is maintained, both groups live in harmony, but the stability of gut flora is very easily upset by many factors – including the persistent administration of antibiotic drugs!

When a baby is born, its digestive tract is completely devoid of micro-organisms. Colonization quickly takes place, however, and the quality and balance of the gut flora which move in will be determining factors in the future health pattern of that individual. A natural inbuilt ability to fight disease by drawing on its own immune strength bodes well for a healthy body and a long life; resorting to antibiotics at the first sign of a cold or a skin problem does not!

The Good Guys

The friendly flora of the digestive tract have many beneficial actions in the healthy activity of the gut and are particularly important in the maintenance of blooming skin. Apart from assisting in the process of detoxification, their natural antibiotic activity helps to boost immunity, inhibit the growth of undesirable bacteria and promote vitamin synthesis.

Repairing the Damage

One of the simplest and safest ways of restoring gut flora balance is to reinstate the beneficial bacteria in the form of live yoghurt and probiotic supplements. Check the label to make sure that the yoghurt and the capsules contain the right kinds of bacteria – *Lactobacillus acidophilus* (which lives in the small intestine) and *Bifido bacterium* (which live in the large bowel). Also, bear in mind that it can take several months to restore the favourable habitat of the intestines (especially after long-term use of antibiotics) and so supplementation may need to be continued for as long as six or even twelve months, accompanied, of course, by a varied and nourishing diet.

Live yoghurt alone is not always sufficient to repopulate the gut after antibiotic ingestion. Whilst good-quality bio-yoghurts are certainly beneficial (their lactic acid content lowers the pH of the intestines and creates a more favourable environment for friendly bacteria to grow), not all the bacteria they contain is likely to survive the rigorous journey through the stomach.

In addition, a number of yoghurts tested for their culture counts were not as 'alive-alive-o' as their packaging proclaimed. Further information on yoghurt can be found on p.36 in the 'Skin Food' section. The chapter on yoghurt in my book *The Food Combining Diet* explains in more detail the different yoghurts which are available.

To encourage re-population of the beneficial bacteria, probiotics in the form of supplements are an invaluable addition. Unfortunately, independent assays carried out around the world have shown that many of the probiotic products on the market simply do not contain the active friendly flora which the labels would suggest. It is therefore vital to choose only those which passed the tests with flying colours. Further information on supplements appears on p.84.

Ask Plenty of Questions

Since antibiotics and other drugs can have a detrimental effect upon the skin and upon the body's systems generally, I always suggest to patients that, if a prescription is proffered, they first ask their medical adviser some pertinent questions, such as:

'What will happen if I refuse your prescription and let the illness/condition take its course?'

'Is my life in danger if I do not take this medication?'

'Am I at risk if I choose to try other, less invasive, treatments before resorting to these antibiotics/steroids/painkillers?'

'What are the likely side effects of the medication you are offering?' ('None' is neither a truthful nor satisfactory answer since all drugs are toxic to a lesser or greater extent.)

'Are you willing to support my decision to delay using these drugs?'

'What are your views, Doctor, on my waiting 24 or 48 hours to see if the illness/condition resolves itself?'

If your G.P. is caring and conscientious, he or she should be sympathetic to your concerns, have no qualms about your capabilities and will be on hand if needed.

ARE DIETARY SUPPLEMENTS REALLY NECESSARY?

In an ideal, unpolluted world, obtaining all the goodness needed from diet alone might be a possibility. That is, of course, so long as that goodness is properly absorbed. Unfortunately, however, the perfect diet has become rather elusive and, in many cases, vitamin and mineral products have become not just a health bonus but an essential requirement.

Here are just a few of the reasons why diet alone may not be enough and where extra nutrients could help:

If you suffer from:

Poor skin, hair or nails
Heavy periods
High blood pressure
High cholesterol
Excessive stress, anxiety or panic attacks
Digestive and/or bowel problems
Persistent colds or other infections

If you:

Smoke
Diet regularly
Drink huge amounts of tea, coffee or cola
Eat lots of sugary or fatty foods
Exist on take-aways or packets and tins
Travel frequently in heavy traffic
Work in a polluted atmosphere
Have been ill
Are waiting for an operation
Are just out of hospital
Are taking regular prescribed or over-the-counter medication, especially HRT, the contraceptive pill or regular doses of aluminium-based indigestion remedies

If you are:

Vegetarian or vegan
Pregnant
Breast-feeding

ARE VITAMIN AND MINERAL SUPPLEMENTS SAFE?

Nutritional supplements have an enviable safety record. Figures produced by the American Centers for Poison Control (they monitor drug safety data) estimate them to be 'at least 1200 times safer than any drug' and, ultimately, following more research 'perhaps tens of thousands of times safer'.

I believe it is unfair and irresponsible to take the view that any one particular method of treatment is better than another. In the same way that drugs are not cure-alls, neither are supplements suitable substitutes for all other treatments. But they are too important to be ignored – or banned in favour of potentially toxic medicines.

Doctors don't have all the answers – and little or no training, experience and understanding of nutrition. There remains an unfortunate tendency to smirch and slander supplements, but a multitude of properly controlled scientific studies carried out around the world continue to show the power and protection that can be provided by natural food substances. Vitamins A, C and E, Essential Fatty Acids, Magnesium, Calcium, Chromium and Selenium are just a few examples of nutrients which have been used in the treatment of a range of medical conditions, from childhood measles, pre-menstrual syndrome and skin disorders to arthritis, heart disease and cancer, with some astonishing and exciting results.

My own experiences, both personally and with patients, have convinced me that top-quality nutrient supplements can be of enormous value in helping to prevent, treat and alleviate many different conditions and are of particular merit in overcoming skin disorders.

But the market is awash with thousands of different products; choosing the right supplements can be a minefield for the unwary. My supplement guidelines may help you to avoid the pitfalls:

- Don't be fooled by cheap products.
- If the label lacks detail, don't buy the product.
- Buy capsules in preference to tablets; fewer nutrients will have been lost during the manufacturing process and there

is no need for the fillers and binders which stick tablets together. The exception to this rule is vitamin B_{12}, which can be destroyed by stomach acids if it is not prescribed as an enteric-coated (protected) tablet.

- The product should be free from gluten, yeast, colours, sugar, lactose, fillers, binders, corn, wheat, salt, preservatives, artificial flavours, milk and soy products (if it is, the label will tell you so); these are often added to save money, they can destroy the nutrients you want and some are potential allergens.

- Be wary of 'kitchen sink supplements' – in other words, those which seem to contain everything but. Products that contain more than 20 ingredients in the same tablet or capsule are unlikely to be of significant benefit.

- Check the sell-by or use-by date.

- Store in a cool, dark place.

- Replace the lid securely after each use.

- Take all supplements with meals unless the label tells you specifically to take them on an empty stomach.

- Be sensible. Follow the pack instructions and never exceed the stated dose. More does not necessarily mean better!

- Don't be frightened by scaremongers who try to persuade you that taking supplements is dangerous or a waste of time. They haven't read the latest research. Good-quality products have an excellent safety record and science has proven them to be of value in fighting free radical damage and treating a wide range of illnesses.

- The word 'supplement' means what it says. Vitamin and mineral capsules should not be viewed as meal replacements and are not substitutes for a nourishing and varied diet.

- There is no need to buy masses of different jars and bottles or lots of separate, isolated nutrients. A good basic supplement programme consists of:

The best quality multivitamin/mineral complex you can afford;

At least one, preferably two grams of vitamin C complex; GLA or evening primrose oil;

Fish oil or linseed oil capsules (if you are not eating oily fish, such as mackerel, trout, sardines and salmon, two or three times per week);

Probiotics are recommended where there has been exposure to antibiotics, in bowel and digestive disorders, poor immune function and where there are skin problems.

Important Note: If you are concerned about your health in any way, please consult your doctor without further delay. Supplements can be enormously helpful but are not substitutes for qualified medical advice. If you are pregnant or are taking regular medication and would like to take supplements as well, it is advisable to let your doctor know.

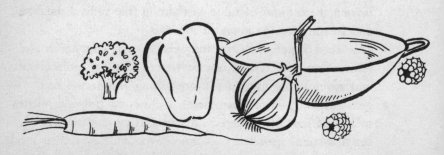

The Importance of Good Digestion

I am convinced digestion is the great secret of life.

Sydney Smith (1771–1845)
English clergyman, essayist and renowned wit

Digestion and Absorption
Eating When You're Hungry
Raw Food
Eating Out
Food Combining

There seems little point in making any effort to improve the quality of food in the diet if no effort is made to improve the quality of digestion and absorption. Otherwise, much beneficial nourishment is likely to be wasted. Healthy skin depends upon a constant supply of top class nutrients – so making sure that those nutrients get to where they are needed is crucially important for skin health.

These tips should help you:

- Make time to eat regular meals, sit down to them and don't leave the table immediately to clear or wash the dishes; rest awhile after eating. Never eat 'on the hoof'.
- Digestion begins in the mouth – that's what your teeth and saliva are for. So take smaller mouthfuls and chew everything thoroughly. The more chewing done by the gnashers, the less churning farther down the tubes and the more efficient the digestion. It sounds like common sense, but how many people do you know who *don't* gulp their food?

- Don't talk with your mouth full. This may seem a ridiculous piece of advice but it is sensible. If you talk whilst you are chewing, you don't chew efficiently – *and* you swallow a lot of air which then rumbles around in the nether regions, interfering with proper digestion!
- Don't drink with meals, except for a small amount which may be required to swallow any supplements or medication.
- Drink plenty of water (preferably filtered) between meals and carry water with you if you are travelling.
- Cut down on tea, coffee and other caffeine-rich drinks such as cola and hot chocolate. Choose herbal or fruit teas, grain-based coffee substitutes, carob drink and fresh fruit juices.
- Don't go for long periods of time without eating. If you know you are likely to miss a meal and will be hungry, take a snack with you and find a quiet spot to settle down and enjoy it without being rushed.
- Keep all fruits and fruit juices away from other foods. Have them as in-between meal snacks and drinks or as a starter but not with a meal – and certainly NEVER after a meal as a dessert.
- When eating out, study the menu carefully and choose items that are naturally lower in fat and not fried or ladled with rich sauces.
- At home, don't deep fry anything. Grill, bake, steam or stir-fry.
- Eat when you are hungry. Don't be forced into food just because the clock tells you it's time to eat.
- Always have breakfast.
- Avoid reheats, except in emergencies. Reheating not only impairs flavour but also disturbs digestion and destroys nutrients. Stored cooked food, even when kept cool, can breed bacteria. If reheating is unavoidable, make sure that

the meal is hot right through before serving and never reheat anything more than once.

- Introduce a small raw salad or selection of crudités 10 to 15 minutes before a cooked meal. The natural enzymes in the raw food help to enhance the digestion of the cooked meal which follows.
- Never eat when stressed, anxious or overtired.
- Wash all fruits and vegetables thoroughly before use and avoid eating fruit skins unless you are sure that they are organically grown.
- Don't eat foods that are very hot or very cold.
- Try to avoid packaged, tinned, convenience and take-away foods which contain excessive amounts of refined flour, refined sugar, salt or spices (e.g. curries, chilli etc.).
- Keep bread and wheat-based cereals to a minimum. Avoid white bread completely.
- Watch out for aluminium in the diet – it can disturb digestion. You'll find it in some kettles, cooking pots and utensils, toothpastes, dried milks, dried soups, coffee creamers, processed cheeses, cartoned juices, cigarette filters, table salt and a wide variety of prescribed medicines, particularly antacid indigestion remedies. Excesses of aluminium can disturb the balance of nutritional minerals in the body such as calcium and magnesium – both essential for healthy skin.
- Set realistic goals for yourself. Don't pursue a particular diet which you hate and which makes you miserable just because you have been told it is good for you.
- Include plenty of variety in your daily diet; be moderate and avoid excesses and extremes.
- Choose food that is as close to its fresh, natural state as possible. In other words, eat food that goes bad – before it goes bad!

- Adopt the easy-to-follow principles set out my book *The Food Combining Diet*, which involves:

  Not mixing starch foods or sugars with proteins at the same meal.

  Keeping fruit away from proteins and starches.

After a few weeks of following this wonderful way of eating, any digestive discomfort should be a thing of the past, absorption and nutrient transport will improve – all vital for helping to improve the health of the skin.

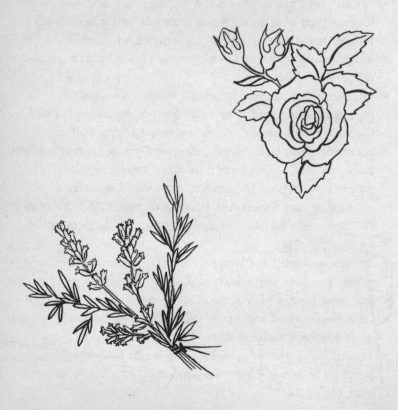

Purity

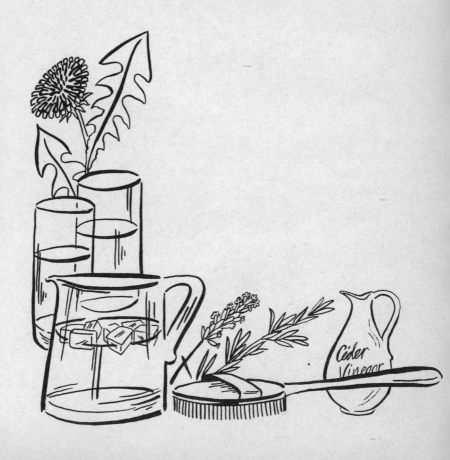

Spring Clean Your Skin, From the Inside . . .

Detoxifying and Cleansing
How Pollution Affects the Skin
Resting the Digestion
Lifting Away the Lethargy
Special Cleansing Diet
Juicing
Wonderful Water

Toxicity is a major handicap to improving skin quality – but invigorating, cleansing skin foods and purifying fluids can scrub your toxic tissues back to life and give your system a completely fresh start. Changing your diet, improving your skin-care routine and allowing your system additional nourishment and protection will help to prevent new build-up.

The human body accumulates poisons from lots of different sources including:

- Prescribed and 'social' drugs
- Cigarette smoke
- Alcohol
- Industrial pollution
- Diet
- Food additives
- Pesticides
- Herbicides
- Fungicides
- Vehicle exhausts
- Internal metabolic wastes

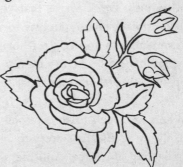

Quite a list, isn't it? The system may appear to cope but is still likely to be stretched to the limits, especially when other stressors are added; for example, anxiety, tension, worry, exhaustion, overwork, missed meals and so on.

When the body is on overload, we may put the red warning signals down to nothing more than 'feeling under par', little realizing that it could take just one more straw to break the camel's back! We are unlikely to be aware of how hard our major routes of elimination – the bowel, bladder and kidneys, the skin itself, the blood and lymph, the R.E.S. (reticulo-endothelial system), lungs, female menstrual flow and liver – are working to keep us healthy and to render the body as free as possible of contamination and pollution.

The liver works particularly hard. A massive filter with over 50 miles of tiny tubing, it screens heavy metals such as aluminium, lead, mercury and cadmium and is responsible for deactivating all the toxic residues from the sources listed on p.95. The only difference between someone who appears to 'get away with it' and another who shows symptoms of toxicity is whether or not the system can cope with the toxic loading without being damaged and still retain sufficient capacity to do other jobs. Don't forget that your poor old liver has also to help control blood glucose, to regulate protein levels, to assimilate fats and control hormonal activity. And when symptoms do begin to develop, they may not necessarily show up on any orthodox medical test scale.

When we reach toxic overload, our skin, hair and nails are likely to be the first areas to register the sapped energy and struggling life force. And the skin takes most of the strain because it is trying desperately to make up for the various inefficiencies of the other overworked organs. Chronic fatigue becomes a wearying nuisance and recurring infections and other illnesses more frequent.

RESTING THE DIGESTION

Spring cleaning the inside also means giving the digestive system a bit of a holiday. Because most bodies are bombarded by constant supplies of food – often processed, refined and full of fats, sugars, salt, spices and stimulants – the digestive system is on permanent overtime. Giving it a rest allows every organ, gland, tissue and cell the chance to relax, unwind, cleanse and recharge.

LIFT AWAY THE LETHARGY!

Choose a couple of days when you are going to be at home and make those cleansing days a regular part of your routine – every two to three weeks. This is my favourite detox diet.

- Rest and relax if you can.
- Go for a walk or spend some time outside in the fresh air – but don't walk or run near fume-laden traffic!
- Practise deep breathing (see p.190).
- Avoid acid-forming foods (e.g. dairy products, meat and bread), keeping mainly to the alkaline-forming fresh vegetables, vegetable juices and fruits which will help to neutralize toxins, speeding their elimination from the body. Clean alkaline-forming foods are easy on the digestion and help to revitalize the blood and tissues. The digestion is rested, the immunity recharged and energy boosted.
- Drink plenty of freshly filtered water throughout the day.

Any headaches, nausea or slight tummy upsets are likely to be signs that the cleansing process is working. Try not to take painkillers or antacids to remove the symptoms of headache or indigestion as drugs put further strain on the liver, encouraging toxins to go back into the tissues and thereby reversing the beneficial elimination process.

If your doctor or hospital has prescribed a special diet (diabetic, for example), or if you are pregnant or on permanent medication for any condition, or if you suffer from an eating disorder such as bulimia or anorexia nervosa, check with your G.P. before following this programme.

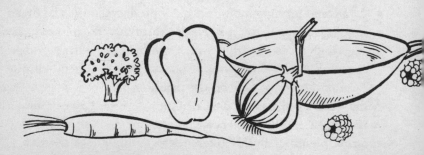

DAY 1

On Waking
Practise the deep breathing exercises set out in the chapter 'Breath of Life', p.190.

On Rising
Begin every day with a glass of boiled, cooled water and a squeeze of fresh lemon juice. It is a wonderful skin cleanser and tonic. Alternatively, enjoy a large cup of herb tea with lemon juice or a glass of filtered water. Or if you have a juicing machine, blend your own favourite combination of fresh fruits.

Breakfast
Choose any fresh fruit and eat as much as you like.

Mid-Morning Break
A cup of herbal tea, glass of fresh juice (not packaged orange juice) or water and a handful of mixed sunflower, pumpkin and sunflower seeds.

Lunch
Large raw vegetable salad containing any ingredients of your choice.

Mid-Afternoon Break
A piece of fruit of your choice. A glass of juice or water if you are thirsty.

Evening Meal

A large portion of steamed or carefully, gently boiled vegetables (take care not to overcook), or any quantity of salad you like.

Before Bed

Small carton of fresh live yoghurt. Or small cup of herb tea or hot Norfolk punch. Supplements if prescribed.

Choose From: Fruits

Apples, apricots (include hunza apricots but avoid dried apricots if they are glazed or preserved), bananas, cherries, blackberries, blueberries, dates, figs, grapefruit, grapes, kiwi fruit, mangoes, nectarines, peaches, pears, pineapple, plums, pumpkin, raspberries.

Salads

Aubergine, avocado, raw beetroot, broccoli florets, cauliflower florets, celery, chicory, cucumber, Chinese leaves, white and red cabbage, grated carrot, courgette, any kind of lettuce, any kind of beans, red or green peppers, any seeds – particularly fenugreek, sesame, sunflower, pumpkin and linseeds, also parsley and other fresh herbs, watercress or fresh sprouts. Add raw onion and garlic if liked.

Other Vegetables

Asparagus, artichokes, any kind of beans, broccoli, bamboo shoots, barley, beet greens, Brussels sprouts, cabbage, calabrese, cauliflower, cauliflower greens, carrots, celeriac, celery, leeks, lentils, marrow, onions, swede, turnips, turnip greens.

DAY 2

For breakfast, lunch and all snacks today use liquids only, choosing a variety of vegetable and fruit juices (preferably prepared at home from fresh produce) – drink any quantity you like. For your evening meal today, include a portion of brown rice with salad or steamed or stir-fried vegetables.

SKIN-SAVING SALAD SUGGESTIONS

Great for your cleansing days but also good starters and snacks for other days too.

- Grated raw beetroot and carrot with chopped onion, parsley and extra virgin olive oil and cider vinegar dressing
- Grated carrot and apple with chopped celery and almonds
- Fenugreek seeds with grated raw garlic, watercress, any grated cabbage, chopped cucumber and pine nuts, dressed with extra virgin olive oil and fresh lemon juice
- Avocado slices with pumpkin seeds
- Sliced apple with dried figs and hazelnuts
- Skinned, sliced tomatoes with chopped basil, parsley and safflower oil
- Broccoli or cauliflower florets dressed with hazelnut oil, cider vinegar and grated Brazils

Remember:

☒ Wash all fruit and vegetables thoroughly before use.
☒ If you feel hungry at any time during the day, don't put up with hunger pangs; enjoy further snacks of more raw vegetables, seeds or fruit or drink vegetable juices.

[X] Don't follow the cleansing routine for more than two or three days at a time or more than once in every two weeks.

[X] Fasting (complete avoidance of food) is not recommended unless you are being supervised by your practitioner. Juice-only diets and fruit diets are common inclusions in women's magazines and can provide a useful (short-term) cleansing programme but should not be followed for more than three days. There is no such thing as a 'juice fast' or a 'fruit fast'. Fasting means taking water only. Unless you are very experienced, fasting without qualified supervision can be extremely dangerous.

FEELING JADED? TRY JUICING

Juicing has recently hit the headlines as 'the latest food phenomenon to sweep America' and is, it seems, all set to do the same in the UK and Europe. But juicing has been around for many, many years and is synonymous with good health and longevity. Daily juicing was the mainstay of famous American naturopaths and physicians such as Benedict Lust and Dr Norman Walker, a recognized authority on nutrition who lived for many hale and hearty years past his century. Some bookshops still carry copies of his classic paperback called *Fresh Vegetable and Fruit Juices* – well worth sleuthing for.

Freshly prepared juices are a real health bonus. Made at home from delicious fruits and vegetables and using a simple juicing machine, they are also great energy boosters and likely to be far more valuable nutritionally than those in bottles or cartons. The regular addition of raw juices to the diet will strengthen body function, providing the body with vital elements for repairing, renewing and revitalizing, encouraging elimination of wastes and improving skin quality. They also have an amazing effect on a sluggish or irritable bowel and can, literally, get you going in the morning!

Juices make a great snack or aperitif and can provide essential nourishment during illness when solid food may not be suitable or acceptable.

All you need to try home-prepared juices for yourself is a juicing machine (available from most good electrical and hardware stores; see also Resources) and lots of fresh fruits and vegetables. Go for fresh fruit juice as a morning wake-up drink or pre-lunch appetizer and a vegetable juice medley prior to the evening meal. For best absorption, take them on an empty stomach – not with the meal. Soon, you'll become really inventive with your recipes, producing colourful and flavourful combinations.

Just wash and peel the fruits and vegetables (no need to peel grapes!), push the pieces into the machine and let the equipment do the rest. In a couple of minutes you'll have a glass of wonderfully energizing fluid packed with vitamins, minerals and natural enzymes.

Go tropical and try fresh pineapple with mango, kiwi and papaya, apple and pear or nectarine with grape. Make a particularly cleansing and tasty aperitif with apple, celery, carrot, grape and beetroot (raw, not cooked!). For more inspiration, look out for *The Complete Raw Juice Therapy* (Thorsons Editorial Board), *A New Way Of Eating* by the *Fit For Life* author Marilyn Diamond and *The Juicing Detox Diet* by Caroline Wheater (Thorsons).

WONDERFUL WATER

'There is no life without water . . . Water is part and parcel of living machinery'. So said Albert von Nagyrapolt Szent-Gyorgi, the man who isolated vitamin C in 1922. Water is essential for skin health and increasing daily consumption of fresh water is beneficial for all skin types. Inadequate water intake can impair every single aspect of our bodily functions. A mere 2 per cent reduction of extra-cellular water can decrease energy levels by as much as one fifth! Too little fluid encourages poor elimination of wastes, can aggravate constipation and lead to urinary tract infections, particularly cystitis.

French surgeon Dr Alexis Carrel was postulating the importance of water as a health-giver in the early 1900s and was awarded the Nobel Prize for Medicine in 1912. 'The cell is immortal', he said. 'It is merely the fluid in which it floats which degenerates. Renew this fluid at proper intervals, give the cells what they require for nutrition and, as far as we know, the pulsation of life may go on forever'.

In 'Fat Facts' and 'Skin Nutrients' we examined the significance and value of the right kinds of fats, oils and fatty acids in achieving and maintaining healthy skin – but without sufficient water, the body is unable to metabolize these important nutrients.

At birth, the human body is made up of 90 per cent water but, on reaching adulthood, this level drops to around 60 per cent. As we age, the body 'tightens', cells begin to suffocate and die in their own waste products, metabolic 'trash' is not eliminated and the lymph system becomes overloaded. Water is needed to dilute the dross and debris so that they can be eliminated from the body. It plays a part in renewing cellular fluids, washing away the garbage and encouraging cell renewal, thereby reducing the effects of wrinkling and ageing.

Filtered water is the best choice; a good-quality filter unit will take out heavy metals such as lead, aluminium and cadmium plus chlorine and nitrates without disturbing the important nutritional minerals such as calcium. Write to manufacturers and seek out independent test results before you buy. Don't rely on the salesman's hype! Water from a good-quality filter is much better and cheaper than bottled water. Use it for cooking and filling the kettle too. Bottled water makes a good standby, especially if you are away from home, but choose those that are labelled 'low sodium': many brands are high in salt, which can disturb potassium balance in the body as well as being drying to the skin.

Try to avoid drinks with meals, apart from the smallest amount needed to swallow any supplements or medication. Too much liquid with food simply makes the stomach contents too dilute; they pass too quickly through the system, digestion is impaired and nutrients are not properly absorbed. A noisy abdomen or 'borborygmus' is a common symptom of a too-liquid meal; the word means flatulence and comes from a Greek word meaning 'I rumble'!

Never drink very hot or very cold liquids: they are too much of a shock to a stomach which evolved before refrigerators, freezers and cookers!

In addition to any juice, coffee, tea or other beverages, try to drink a litre of water (approximately two pints) each day. This isn't difficult if you have a glass of water 10 to 15 minutes before each meal and keep another glass nearby to sip at during the day. At work, give the vending machine a miss and drink water instead. Excessive amounts of coffee and tea overtax the liver and kidneys and rob the body of nutritional minerals; but unless your skin problem is very severe, or food tests show them to be a factor, it shouldn't be necessary to give up tea and coffee altogether. Quality tea and coffee is often lower in caffeine than the cheaper varieties. Small amounts – say one to three cups daily – can be beneficial. (See Resources.) If you are trying to cut down on tea and coffee, experiment with herbal teas, grain-based coffee substitutes, dandelion coffee, juices or savoury herbal drinks.

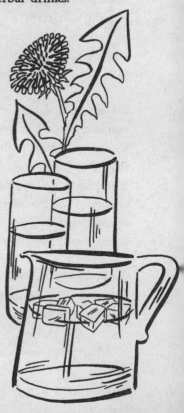

. . . And From the Outside!

Bath twice a day to be really clean, once a day to be passably clean, once a week to avoid being a public menace.

Anthony Burgess (b. 1917), *Inside Mr Enderby*, 1963

> Cleansing
> Skin Airing
> Skin Brushing
> Exfoliation
> Save the Soap
> Bath-Time Beauty
> Essential Oils
> Cellulite
> Salt Bathing

Cleaning the outside skin isn't just down to cleansing lotions or soap and water. You owe yourself more than that. Real cleansing means preventing those pores from choking to death, sloughing off dead cells and eliminating impurities, allowing the skin to 'breathe' and renew itself more efficiently. Don't forget that the skin, along with the bowel, bladder, kidneys, lungs and lymph system, is an important 'organ of elimination' and that when one area is sluggish, the others will try to share the load. So by making sure that the skin is functioning properly, other parts of the body will begin to work more efficiently too.

SKIN AIRING

Apart from in the height of summer or when we are holidaying in a warm climate, our skins tend to remain well covered. But airing the skin daily helps to regulate body temperature and improve circulation.

An 'old-fashioned' method of exposing the skin to fresh air is quoted almost lyrically by the famous 1930s fitness expert Mrs Mary M. Bagot Stack in her book called *Building The Body Beautiful - The Bagot Stack Stretch and Swing System* - now a collector's item. 'First thing, then,' she tells us, 'every morning, spring out of bed before you have time to hesitate or start that long line of thought which leads nowhere; throw open the windows. At first wear a bathing-dress and five jumpers if you feel the cold. But as your circulation improves each day, wear less and less, until finally your last bit of discarded silk or muslin can go across the window, for the sake of the neighbours but not around you!' Mrs Bagot Stack's suggestions of more than half a century ago may seem amusing and quaint but were followed by millions of dedicated ladies at the time. Gatherings of 10,000 or more - all in the appropriate workout gear of the day - followed her exercise and breathing directions at regular rallies in London's Hyde Park.

Allowing unclothed skin to 'air' and practising your deep breathing exercises, especially near an open window, really will help to kick-start a sleepy body in the morning. It takes courage to begin with but the long term benefits are really worthwhile, especially if you are likely to be spending the rest of the day indoors!

BATHING

The word which usually springs to mind when we talk about the need for bathing or showering is 'cleanliness'. But a little extra time spent in the bath or shower than our usual daily dash can bring with it enormous health benefits and improvements to skin quality too.

In the early 1900s, keeping clean was not so simple. Public bathing was more commonplace than it is now, each public bath (in London, at least) serving around 2000 people! Few houses had indoor plumbing and where a bathroom was boasted, it was usually of the cold comfort variety. But most modern dwellings have bathrooms luxurious enough to make relaxation a pleasure. So if you are an 'in-and-outer', slow down. Your health and your skin could benefit.

SKIN BRUSHING

Brushing the hair is normal enough but, if you have never heard of it before, brushing the skin can seem a strange suggestion – until you realize what good sense it makes.

The health of the skin is determined to a great degree by its ability to repair and replace itself. If dead cells are not removed, pores can become clogged and congested. Where elimination is sluggish, new cells cannot work their way to the surface – or may not be manufactured in the first place – and so damaged skin cannot heal. Whilst skin cells are shed constantly (90 per cent of all household dust is said to be discarded human skin particles!), skin brushing stimulates the process into more efficient action. Circulation is improved, impurities are released and skin is healthier and softer.

The best and most effective skin brushes are made from natural materials and are usually used dry, before bathing. However, some ultra-sensitive skins may be more suited to wet brushing or to a loofah or bath mitt.

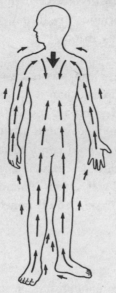

Focus your movements towards the heart. Work your way from the soles of the feet, up the legs (remembering to brush the back of them as well as the front), over the thighs, buttocks, hips and torso, then up the arms towards the shoulders. Avoid the face but include the back of the neck. However, don't strain to reach the inaccessible parts of your back. And be gentle!

Other Effective Exfoliators

If brushing is difficult for you or, for some reason, not possible, stroke the skin firmly with an old and rough flannel face cloth, dry or wet. Damp cosmetic sponges (use a clean one each time) are good for the facial skin and can be used with cleansers, scrubs and moisturizers. Or choose a body scrub cream or lotion which you can massage into wet skin and rinse off in the bath or shower. A further option is to use a handful of sea salt (although not suitable for dry skin) with a few drops of lavender or tea tree essential oil added. Massaged into the skin before bathing or showering, this combination detoxifies and cleanses. If you use the salt without the oil, then make sure to moisturize the skin after washing.

For very hard skin – on the heels for example – rub with dry or wet oat bran. If your skin is so sensitive that it even reacts to the word 'hypoallergenic', try a mixture of organic oatmeal and a few drops of chamomile or juniper essential oil.

How Often?

After you have been skin brushing for a few weeks, you will recognize automatically when it needs to be done. Since the gentle friction of brushing, loofahing and scrubbing actually cleanses the skin, I would recommend it every two to three days if you are showering or bathing every day. Brush every day if you shower or bathe less often than this.

WHICH IS BETTER – SHOWER OR BATH?

If you can, alternate between the bath and the shower. Showers tend to be stimulating (good for bringing you round in the morning) and baths are best for winding down. Tepid showers are great if you need to be really alert (especially after a late night!) but don't take very cold showers if you have a heart condition or high or low blood pressure.

BATH-TIME BEAUTY PROTECTION PLAN

- If you are skin brushing for the first time, start off with a flannel or loofah mitt (used wet) and progress to a skin brush after a few weeks. Don't brush where the skin is broken. Brushing is helpful before and after hair removal to prevent ingrowing hairs.
- Avoid bubble baths, which are usually made from strong detergents.
- Avoid ordinary tablets of soap, which are alkaline and disturb the skin's natural acid mantle. If you are an enthusiastic soap fan, choose a non-alkaline (natural or balanced pH) cleansing bar instead.
- Use a battery or electric shaver rather than a wet blade for de-fuzzing – better for sensitive skins and no risk of cuts.
- If you can't live without bubbles in the bathwater, run a capful of moisturizing shampoo under the tap – it doesn't strip the skin of natural oils like bubble baths and washing-up liquids.
- If you suffer with skin redness or irritation, try adding cider vinegar to the bath water; it restores the natural pH (see the Appendix, 'First Aid For Skin').
- If your skin is very dry, add a couple of tablespoons of virgin olive oil to the water and soak for ten minutes. Don't use any soap or cleansers. The oil acts as an emulsifier which picks up debris so you will remove any impurities when you rub yourself dry.
- Skin brushes, loofahs, flannels and towels should be washed regularly; if possible, every day. They pick up an enormous amount of bacteria and dead skin with each use.
- If you are over-tired or stressed, make a relaxing potion with an infusion (just as you would make tea) of rosemary and lavender, dried or fresh, and pour it into the bath

water. Some stores now sell herbal sachets especially for bath time but just as useful (and often less expensive) are the herbal teabags in the kitchen cupboard. Just pop one into the bath while the water is running. It's not a good idea to place fresh or dried herbs directly into the bath as they can block the plug hole or drain.

- Don't soak in the bath for longer than 20 minutes – especially if your skin tends to be dry.

- Don't have the bath or shower too hot. This can encourage broken surface veins, may put unnecessary strain on the heart and will destroy the skin's protective acid mantle. It can also contribute to premature skin ageing, for skin cells age more quickly as the temperature of the body rises. Generally when our bodies heat up – for example, during hard physical work – they produce sweat, which not only rids the body of toxins but also cools the blood near the skin surface as it evaporates, then allowing blood from deeper tissues to carry heat out to the surface. But when we are immersed in a hot bath, for example, a hot tub or even relaxing in a sauna, the body cannot cool itself properly and cellular ageing speeds up.

- After-bath body lotions, moisturizers and oils will be absorbed more effectively by damp, just-washed skin. Pay particular attention to knees, elbows, thighs, ankles, heels and hands.

- Shower gels are less drying than straightforward soap but do make sure you rinse them away thoroughly.

- If you use bath oils, remember that the bath will be much more slippery – so take care!

THE VALUE OF ESSENTIAL OILS

An expert aromatherapy massage can stimulate, relax, cleanse and heal. If you can afford to, treat yourself to this sheer delight once a month. And don't forget how therapeutic essential oils can be in the home. Geranium is restorative and balancing; juniper is particularly cleansing; rosemary helps oily skin and combines well with juniper; lavender is calming and relaxing but also uplifting; both tea tree and lemon oils are detoxifying. The combinations and uses are myriad. Put a few drops in the bath water or into a base oil massaged into your skin before bathing or showering.

This is my favourite detox massage combination (which also seems to help hormonal imbalances and fluid retention):
50ml base oil (I prefer to use extra virgin olive oil, almond oil, or grapeseed oil which is odourless)
5 drops each of geranium, juniper, lavender and rosemary

For expert information on the use of essential oils, check the Recommended Reading list on p.214.

THE CELLULITE SOLUTION!

Is it my imagination but did anyone ever bother about cellulite before bikinis and cutaway swimsuits? Whilst many doctors still pursue the line that there is no such thing as cellulite, it remains an indisputable fact of female life – and affects fatties and skinnies alike. Inaccurately named during the last century, cellulite was once believed (mistakenly) to be a type of inflammatory condition ('cellule' meaning 'of the cell' and 'ite' indicating 'inflammation').

Cellulite is, in fact, fatty 'tissue sludge'. Hormonal changes (brought about by puberty, pregnancy, the contraceptive pill or the menopause) encourage fat cells to become interspersed with fluid. The delicate mechanism which would normally push blood and nutrients to the cells and extract wastes from them is disturbed. The fat cells become enlarged and waterlogged, compressing the capillaries; circulation slows down and the skin takes on an 'orange peel' appearance. The bumpy goose flesh is often cold to the touch and, although it can appear on any part of the body, is most common to the hips, thighs, buttocks, upper arms and, occasionally, the abdomen. What all these areas have in common is lack of movement, so it makes sense that to reduce cellulite, you must increase circulation.

Poor lymph drainage, stress (which can have a detrimental effect upon hormones), bad posture, lack of exercise and junk diets add to the problem. So, too, do tobacco, excessive caffeine-laden beverages or alcohol; all bad habits likely to spread, rather than shed, stubborn cellulite.

Anti-Cellulite Action

A combination of regular massage, detoxification, exercise, improved circulation and a nutrient-dense diet are the keys to banishing cellulite.

Move! Too much sitting or standing slows the circulation. Take a brisk 10 minute walk every day or 20 to 30 minutes two or three times a week. If the weather is inclement (or it's dark and, perhaps, not safe to venture outside), then make regular use of a rebounder (mini-trampoline); great for detoxifying, shedding dead skin cells and improving blood flow. Ten or fifteen minutes rebounding (you don't need high ceilings or special clothing) is equivalent to half an hour's hard slog on the tarmac but without jarring the spine.

Exfoliate and Stimulate

Regular exfoliation is essential in the crusade against cellulite, so use that skin brush or loofah mitt! Add lavender, lemon and cypress oils (two drops each) either to the bath water or mix with almond oil as a carrier and massage into the skin before bathing. If possible, shower or splash with tepid water when you emerge from the bath. After your cool rinse, use the same oil mixture and rub into the affected areas.

Diet Makes a Definite Difference

If you are a cellulite sufferer, then the cleansing day diet is essential. So, too, are additional fluids. Drink plenty of water – four to six glasses per day – and try fennel, fenugreek, sage and vervain teas which are detoxifying and cleansing. Vitamin C, bioflavonoids and vitamin E are great anti-cellulite supporters so the diet should include lots of fresh fruits, vegetables, nuts and seeds with extra help from supplements (see chapter entitled 'Skin Nutrients').

Cleansing herbs such as dandelion, burdock, sarsaparilla and yellow dock, with their natural diuretic and detoxifying properties are a useful addition to an anti-cellulite diet. Dandelion is rich in minerals and is a natural diuretic and liver decongestant. Burdock improves lymph drainage and therefore reduces internal toxicity. It also neutralizes poisonous wastes and stimulates kidney and liver function. Old herbal folklore recommends burdock as specific for skin eruptions and inflammation as in eczema, psoriasis and urticaria. Sarsaparilla is a first class acne remedy, its benefits possibly being related to its hormone-balancing action and ability to remove bacteria. Yellow dock helps reduce inflammation, particularly of the lymph glands, and has a history of use in soothing nettle rash. In herbal cleansing remedies, these four powerful blood cleansers are often to be found in combination.

Important Note: Unless you are being advised by a qualified medical herbalist, herbal remedies are best taken in the form of brand-named tablets, from health-food stores or good chemists, which state clearly the recommended dosage. Home preparation of raw herbs should be left to those with experience.

SALT BATHS

In cases of severe toxicity, soaking in hot salt water will encourage perspiration and draw potentially harmful toxins out through the pores of the skin.

Add 1lb (approx. 1/2 kg) of Epsom salts or ordinary household salt into a bath of comfortably hot water. Immerse the body up to the neckline and stay put for no less than 10 minutes but no more than 20.

Take your salt bath once a week either last thing at night immediately before going to bed or, if during the day, go to bed for approximately two hours afterwards.

Do not rinse the body but pat yourself dry with a warm towel.

Put on warm, comfortable nightwear and go straight to bed, keeping yourself well covered.

Upon rising, rinse yourself thoroughly with tepid water (shower if possible) and follow with a vigorous rub down with a clean dry towel.

Note: The cleansing effects of salt bathing may cause mild dizziness or slight nausea for a short while. Getting out of a hot bath can also cause a temporary lowering of blood pressure. It is therefore wise to get out slowly and sit down on a chair for a minute or two before drying off. If you have limited movement or have been ill it is advisable to have a family member or partner close at hand.

Salt bathing is not suitable for anyone with blood pressure, heart or kidney problems unless medically supervised.

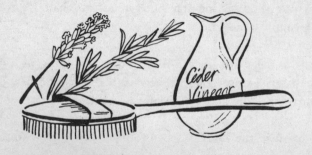

THREE

Beauty

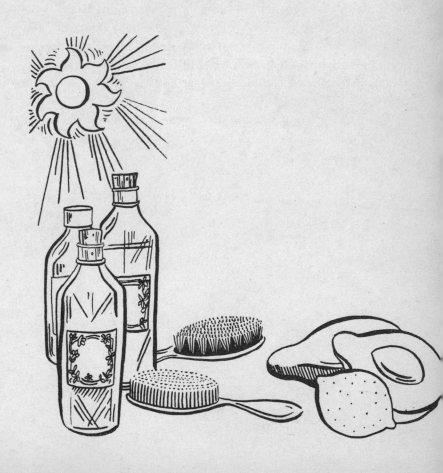

Caring For Your Skin Type

As a white candle
In a holy place
So is the beauty
Of an aged face.

Joseph Campbell (c. 1881-1944), Irish poet

Dry Skin
Sensitive Skin
Oily Skin
Combination Skin
Day Care
Night Nourishment
Scrubs, Steaming and Face Packs
Soap
Aromatherapy Facial

Basic skin type is determined by genetic disposition and will usually have become apparent by the age of 12 or 13. But it can also be influenced by a range of other factors too, including diet, environment, stress threshold, how well we digest and absorb our food and the cosmetics and skin-care products we use. Skin condition may also be affected by illness, fluctuating hormone levels, changes in the weather, lack of exercise, anxiety and trauma and, of course, by age, tending to become drier as we grow older. A lack of oil is not, in itself, a cause of skin dryness. Both oily and combination skins can lack moisture.

Most people know their skin type but if you are unsure, the following pointers should help.

DRY SKIN

- Flaky patches
- Chaps easily
- Feels tight, especially across the cheeks, forehead and chin
- Prone to itching and irritation

Dryness is exacerbated by exposure to detergents, central heating, air conditioning systems, smoky, polluted atmospheres, inadequate skin care, poor diet and overexposure to the sun. Check your current cleanser, moisturizer and night cream. Are they right for your skin type or could they be too drying? Given proper attention and the right internal and external care, dry skin can be normalized and encouraged to retain more moisture.

Never leave the skin unprotected. After cleansing with a creamy or milky lotion or oil, wipe away any excess with a damp cotton pad, rinse with tepid water, pat dry (use a toner if you like, too) and, immediately, apply moisturizer. Water does not dehydrate dry skin except when used with harsh alkaline soaps. A water rinse helps to improve circulation and encourages the moisturizer to be absorbed more efficiently into the skin's surface. Always pat dry before applying moisturizer.

Skin products containing the following herbs may help dry skin: arnica, chamomile, cucumber, evening primrose oil, eyebright, lavender, linden blossom, marsh mallow.

Jojoba and almond oils are great for massaging dry skin and are also effective make-up removers.

SENSITIVE SKIN

- Reddens easily
- Subject to broken capillaries
- Aggravated by ordinary soap
- High cheek colour
- Prone to itching and irritation

Ultra-sensitivity is a real nuisance and can apply to any skin type. Reduce adverse reactions by calming and strengthening the skin both from the inside and the outside. Eat plenty of healing skin foods and add an evening primrose oil or GLA supplement to your diet. A good-quality multivitamin/mineral complex and extra vitamin C are also excellent sensitive-skin supporters. Choose high-quality hypoallergenic skin-care products which are designed especially for your skin type. Always ask for samples of any new products so that you can test for sensitivity before buying larger sizes. The list at the back of the book should help you.

OILY SKIN

- Overall shine
- Visible open pores
- Coarse texture
- Tends to 'shed' powder and foundation
- Prone to spots and blackheads
- Poor circulation
- Sallow complexion

Don't be tempted to attack oily skin with drying, astringent lotions. The sebaceous glands will simply overreact by producing more oil. Some experts are adamant that toners should be avoided by all skin types but I have found them to be valuable if used in the right circumstances. Astringent lotions and toners cannot 'close' the pores. They act by plumping the skin slightly to give it a more even-textured appearance. Flooding an open-pored skin with toner may make matters worse if pores are clogged but, otherwise, can be useful for removing excess cleanser, for freshening and for hastening the departure of troublesome whiteheads and boils. Toners assist in strengthening that all-important acid mantle and also help to moisturize the skin by enhancing the absorption of creams and oils, so they are useful for dry as well as for greasy skins.

Apply a lightweight moisture lotion (one designed for oily skin) after cleansing and toning. Skin products containing the following herbs may help oily or blemished skin: aloe vera, birch, burdock, ivy, calendula, chestnut, horsetail, witch hazel.

Oily and blemished skin is dealt with in more detail in the chapter 'Acne Attack', p.136.

COMBINATION SKIN

- Oily 'T' zone over forehead, nose, sides of nose and chin
- Normal or dry on cheeks
- Prone to blemishes

As with oily skin, overexposure to harsh treatments can make the oily 'T' panel more active. I have found the best way to care for combination skin is to treat it as normal, by following the Common-Sense Skin Schedule.

COMMON-SENSE SKIN SCHEDULE

The following skin-care routine is suitable for most skin types (oily and blemished skins should turn to p.143). However, although fitting into basic categories, everyone's skin has its own characteristics so feel free to adapt my suggestions to your own needs. Just remember not to overcleanse, overstimulate, overscrub or overmoisturize.

In the same way that you enjoy a change of scene or a different outfit, skin will benefit if you ring the product changes. When buying skin-care creams and lotions, find at least two 'sets' which suit your skin type and alternate them. Use one set of cleanser, toner and moisturizer for your morning routine and a different group at night. Daytime skin care is all about protection – against pollution and dehydration. At night, skin needs to rest and regenerate. It's no use relying on just one cream to do both jobs – so choose products which will support your skin's needs during waking and sleeping.

Night-Time Clean Up

Remove eye make-up with a gentle eye cleanser. (Ordinary skin cleansers are not always 'active' enough to remove heavy or waterproof eye make-up and, in addition, can sometimes make the eyes sore.) Then use a quality cold-pressed oil (or your own favourite cleanser) and, with clean fingers, massage a small amount well into the skin for several minutes. Remove any excess with damp cotton pads (not tissues, they're too harsh).

Tone Up
Rinse the face with cool water and pat dry with a clean towel.

Soften Up
Choose a night moisturizer suitable for your skin type and massage a small amount over the whole of the face – avoiding

the eye area which should be treated with special eye cream. Over-use of night creams, particularly around the eyes, can cause puffiness. Don't forget to pay extra special attention to the neck, too (see p.182).

Morning Cleanse

Use a soap-free facial wash or a cleansing lotion and massage into damp skin. Remove excess with cotton pads or rinse with warm water. (Your cleanser should be different from the one you used last night.)

Tone

Complete all rinsing routines with a cold water splash and pat dry.

Nourish

Use a protective day moisturizer and follow with your usual make-up routine.

POWDERS

Use translucent loose powder to set your make-up base and give that professional finishing touch. Keep compressed powder for touching up only. Remember to change powder pads and puffs regularly. They hang on to dead skin cells and breed bacteria. An alternative to compressed powder are those tiny paper sheets (in miniature book form) which are impregnated with powder. They are hygienic and lightweight; they fit easily into make-up purse, handbag or pocket and there's no risk of spillage. Just tear out a new page each time.

SCRUBS

I have heard some experts advise against the use of exfoliating scrubs and peeling creams, believing that they are too harsh for some skins and expose new cells prematurely. Whilst this may be acceptable advice for normal skins which behave as they should, this has not been my own experience. Oily and blemished skins need that extra stimulus to shed surface debris and scrubs do a great job in improving circulation, skin tone and clarity.

Treat your skin firmly but gently when using exfoliating products. Choose a scrub suited to your skin type and use it once a week if your skin is dry and two or three times per week for greasy complexions.

If your skin is ultra-sensitive, coarse-grained scrubs can intensify the condition. On the other hand, improving circulation nearly always helps to make it less so. However, if you find all scrubs too harsh, massage gently with a cosmetic sponge or face cloth when you cleanse and wash.

STEAMING

Water vapour is very cleansing and makes skin more receptive to cleansers, moisturizers and packs. Water also plumps the skin and helps to reduce fine lines and wrinkles. Regular steaming is relaxing and soothing. It improves circulation, cleanses deep down and softens the skin. Before treatment, protect any tiny red surface veins with a squeeze of vitamin E from a capsule or with a little vitamin E cream.

For dry or normal skins, treat yourself to a facial sauna once or twice a month. If the skin is oily, then steam it more often (see p.146).

Begin by removing all traces of make-up with your usual cleanser. Wipe away any excess but don't splash with cold water or use toner at this stage. Lean over a basin of just-boiled water or use a facial sauna unit (one or two minutes for dry, sensitive and normal skins; four or five minutes for oily skins). After steaming, blot away excess moisture by pressing an opened-out tissue gently over the face.

FACE PACKS

Whilst the skin is still warm and damp, apply a mask suitable for your skin type; either your own favourite purchase or a home-made version. Reapply a little vitamin E cream or oil to any sore skin or broken veins and avoid these areas when applying the mask.

Dry and mature skins respond well to a mixture of avocado, honey and sour cream or mashed banana mixed with beaten egg. Masks for oily skin are on p.147. Mix equal parts of the ingredients together and spread over cleansed skin, avoiding the eye area. Cover the eyes with squeezed-out herbal teabags or damp cotton pads soaked in herbal eyebright solution or witch hazel. Relax for 10 to 15 minutes. Rinse the mask with tepid water, splash with cool water, pat dry and then apply moisturizer as usual, not forgetting the neck.

SOAP AND THE ACID MANTLE

Many people are set in their soap and water ways but it's worth knowing that not all soap is a skin's best friend. Soreness, irritation, redness, even attacks of thrush and cystitis, can be aggravated by the wrong kinds of soap products, particularly if they contain harsh chemicals, colourings, deodorants, lanolin, perfumes and detergents (which may not always be immediately apparent from the product name or packaging).

Due to its alkaline nature, using soap, especially around the genital and anal areas, will upset the body's natural ecology and skin's pH, destroying the acid mantle, leaving the skin unprotected and lacking in natural moisture. Although the normal slightly acid state would, under the right circumstances, be restored within a few hours, it is likely to be wiped out quickly by yet more soaping. Moisturizing non-alkaline soap bars, liquid soaps and cleansing emulsions are more gentle on the skin.

Whilst it is always sensible to check with your doctor if you have a skin problem, many inflammations and irritations are caused simply by over-washing with the wrong products. Where the diet lacks essential fatty acids, the skin is also likely to suffer more from allergic reactions since there is less natural protection available.

AROMATHERAPY FACIAL

Treat your skin to a cleansing, nourishing and revitalizing facial using pure essential oils. The gentle, soothing massage not only promotes relaxation but also improves circulation and leads to firmer skin, by strengthening and toning the underlying muscle tissue. Be sure to use only unadulterated oils – synthetics are *not* an adequate alternative – and follow the dilution instructions carefully.

Cleanse
Add 3 drops of a purifying oil such as rosemary, lavender or peppermint (or a blend) to 1 teaspoon of almond oil and massage into your skin to remove dirt, bacteria and make-up. Rinse with warm (not hot) water.

Facial Steam
A facial steam opens pores and releases impurities. Fill a large bowl with just-boiled water and add 10 drops of essential oil. Drape a towel over your head to keep in the steam and hold your face over the bowl for five minutes.

Scrub
Exfoliate to remove dead skin cells and unclog pores. Use one of the following combinations:

- For oily skin: make a paste by mixing 1 tablespoon of corn meal with honey, then add 3 drops of lavender, lemon, ylang ylang or geranium oil.
- For acne: make a paste by mixing 1 tablespoon of corn meal with honey, then add 3 drops of juniper, lavender, tea tree (see page 147) or bergamot oil.
- For dry or mature skin: make a paste by mixing 1 tablespoon of almond meal with honey, then add 3 drops of rose, sandalwood, geranium or chamomile oil.

Massage the paste gently into your skin for a few minutes, then rinse with warm water.

Facial Mask

Prepare a facial mask with one of the following combinations:

- For oily skin or acne: mix 1 tablespoon of clay (from health food shops) with ½ teaspoon of honey and 3 drops of lavender or tea tree oil.
- For dry and mature skin: mix 1 tablespoon of oat bran with ½ teaspoon of honey and 3 drops of rose or geranium oil.

Apply the mask to the face and neck, taking care to avoid the eye area. Soak cotton pads in rose or lavender water (not in undiluted oil) and place over the eyes. Lie down, with your feet slightly higher than your head, and relax for a quarter of an hour, perhaps listening to soothing music. Then rinse off the mask with warm water and gently pat dry.

Tone

Make a toner by mixing 1 drop of geranium or lavender oil with 8fl oz (230ml) of distilled water. Shake before use. Soak a cotton ball and smooth over your face and neck.

Moisturize

To complete the facial, apply a nourishing moisturizer made by adding 10 drops of your favourite essential oil to 1fl oz (35ml) of base oil such as almond, grapeseed or sunflower. Place 3 drops of the mixture in your hand, add several drops of floral water or spray (see below) and massage into your face.

Facial Spray

To replenish the water lost from your skin throughout the day, spray regularly with a floral spray made of 5 drops of lavender, rose, sage or rosemary oil (or a blend) added to 8fl oz (230ml) of distilled water, stored in a spray bottle. Shake before use.

Safe in the Sun

Natural forces are the healers of disease.

Hippocrates (c. 460 – 377 BC), Greek physician and founder of the
Hippocratic school of medicine.

Vitamin D
Sunbathing
Heatstroke and Sunburn
Sun Skin Care
Sunless Bronzers

We are so confused by conflicting reports about the benefits
and dangers of sun exposure that it can be impossible to
decide whether to stay inside or enjoy the great outdoors. One
news item will caution against sun bathing because of the risk
of skin cancer whilst another tells us that going out in the sun
reduces the likelihood of this devastating disease.

As with so many things in life, the Arndt-Schulz law
(established in 1880) applies: 'Small doses stimulate, moderate
doses inhibit, large doses kill.'

Short periods of time in the sun are positively beneficial. Some
ultra-violet light is essential for our well-being and regular but
sensible amounts appear actually to reduce the risk of cancer.
Body rhythms, hormone levels, vitamin D production and
calcium absorption are all controlled by the action of daylight
picked up by the eyes and transmitted to the pineal gland
(situated in the brain and known as the seat of the soul and
vestigial remnant of the 'third eye'). Calcium is one of the
nutrients which help to prevent uncontrolled growth of cancer

cells and research is continuing which may show vitamin D to be of similar value.

You could say that the pale-skinned inhabitants of Northern European extraction actively encourage the risk of cancer by indulging in extreme behaviour. They stay almost completely covered all year only to throw caution to the winds during a couple of vacation weeks in high summer, when they turn out in the briefest of bikinis on to a burning beach. The pursuit of a 'holiday tan at any cost' clouds common sense. It's when we are exposed to sunburning (as opposed to sunlight) that danger manifests.

It was once thought that only UVB rays, which are held responsible for tanning and sunburn, caused damage to the skin, while the UVA rays, which do not burn the skin, were relatively harmless – but new evidence suggests that UVA rays may, in fact, be just as harmful. UVA rays are now held to penetrate the skin more deeply and to cause greater long-term damage to skin elasticity. So, just because you don't burn, doesn't mean you have avoided sun damage altogether; to minimize skin aging wear a moisturizer with a built-in sunscreen, even on overcast days. And be aware that sun beds, while they do not burn the skin, emit mostly UVA rays.

One thing is for certain. Too much sun makes the skin tough, lined and leathery; well, it's not called 'tanning' for nothing! Baking your bare bits without the protection of moisturizing sun lotions and oils is just plain impetuous. Whilst mahogany hues are passé, market research polls show that few people are happy to remain pasty and pale. It seems that a tan boosts morale and confidence, and makes us feel healthier and more positive.

Here's how to benefit from the sun's health-giving properties and protect yourself from damage at the same time:

- Get outside during all weathers. Skin health will benefit even on an overcast day.
- If you are going for that golden tán, build up sun exposure gradually over a period of several weeks before the holiday (10–15 minutes a day before 11am or after 3pm).
- Never sunbathe between 12 noon and 2.30 pm. The sun's rays are strongest and most damaging during this period.
- Never fall asleep in the sun.
- Choose a sun protection lotion or cream which suits your skin type and re-apply it throughout the day, especially after swimming or if you've become hot and sweaty. Use a sun block and protective balm on your lips. Be careful when buying products abroad; American and European Sun Protection Factors and UVA/UVB ratings are not always the same.
- If you suffer from a rash as a result of being out in the sun, try changing your sun lotion before you blame the sun itself. Some products, even if labelled 'hypoallergenic', can cause this painful and unpleasant reaction. Blisters and boils can be triggered by certain drugs. Several patients have reported skin eruptions after sun exposure which have, subsequently, been linked to prescribed and over-the-counter medications. Don't assume that medicine residues are always passed out of the body. Although quite rare, it seems that antibiotics, anti-inflammatory medicines, diuretics, tranquillizers or the contraceptive pill taken within the previous two years can still cause a flare-up!
- At the end of a day in the sun, apply after-sun moisture lotion or gel to guard against wrinkles and drying. Don't forget to look after your hands and feet too.
- Take care if sunbathing near to water, snow or ice. The light

reflected from them will intensify the effect of UV rays. And you'll need greater protection the nearer you travel to the equator or the higher you go up a mountain!

- Don't neglect your normal skin-care routine. Keep up with the skin brushing, massage and moisturizing and your tan will last longer.
- Eat plenty of antioxidant-rich fresh fruits and vegetables and drink lots of water. This applies throughout the year but is especially important if you are a regular sun worshipper.
- Take a top-quality antioxidant supplement which contains vitamins C, E, beta carotene and selenium – as well as either evening primrose oil or GLA – every day to give additional protection against free radical damage and help keep skin healthy and supple.
- If your skin is the type that never tans or if photosensitivity prevents your going out in the sun – but you'd like to have a tan just the same – try a sunless bronzer. They are also useful for colouring the skin before a holiday or special event which demands sleeveless, low cut or skin-revealing clothing. Technological advances mean that these useful artificial tanning creams have lost their ersatz orange pigment and their ominous odour. These days, no-one will guess the difference.
- Where the sun is very hot, always wear a hat. If you are unlucky enough to be affected by sunstroke or heatstroke, drink lots of water and fresh juices, eat extra fresh fruit and take 2 grams of vitamin C every four hours until symptoms subside. Bach Rescue Remedy and Homoeopathic Arnica are also useful.
- For sunburn, follow the treatment for heatstroke and apply vitamin E (break open capsules) four times daily; as long as the skin is unbroken, also spread the affected area with plain live yoghurt.

135

Acne Attack

Dermatology is the best speciality. The patient never dies – and never gets well.

Anonymous

Antibiotics – and Probiotics
Hormones
Good Digestion
Foods to Avoid
Skin-Care Routine
Case History

DEALING WITH ACNE AND OILY SKIN

Acne vulgaris is a condition most commonly associated with the teenage years and early twenties. The name sounds just about as disheartening as the condition itself, which causes untold misery to millions of youngsters just at a time in their lives when they are striving to look their best. Interestingly, in 'developed' nations, acne is believed to afflict around 75 per cent of all teenagers to a greater or lesser degree but in underdeveloped countries, where processed foods are unknown and junk diets don't exist, acne is not a problem.

It is this single fact which, for me, makes the commonly held medical view that diet has no effect on acne so surprising. Lack of exercise, the officials say, 'is not a factor as far as we know' and 'lack of hygiene is not to blame either'. Yet exercise, by improving circulation and assisting detoxification, does seem to help. And proper cleansing certainly assists in reducing inflammation and cross-infection.

THE ORTHODOX VIEW

'Official' literature recommends the use of Benzoyl peroxide, an anti-bacterial agent with known side effects such as soreness, irritation and excessive dryness.

In addition, hydrocortisone creams are often suggested, but can thin and waste the skin with prolonged use. Topical and oral antibiotics have a range of side effects including bacterial resistance, thrush and diarrhoea. Oral hormones work to reduce the levels of testosterone, the male hormone believed to be responsible for the higher-than-average sebum production (the skin's own natural oil) so common in acne sufferers. But is it really safe or sensible to administer hormones by mouth to a youngster whose own hormones are already wildly out of balance? It's well known that, whilst the contraceptive pill can reduce acne in some cases, it is also responsible for causing it in others.

One senior dermatologist is quoted as saying that 'antibiotics remain central to therapy because doctors are used to them and because they are cheap'. At the same time, he confirmed that persistent doses of antibiotics cause side effects which include a range of gastrointestinal disorders, e.g. indigestion, constipation, irritable bowel syndrome and candidiasis as well as persistent and recurring infections.

Retin A, a drug which contained high doses of vitamin A, was routinely prescribed for severe cases of acne until it was discovered that one of its side effects was to cause deformity in foetuses.

The common denominator in all these orthodox 'remedies' is that they attack only the symptoms and do nothing to alleviate the cause of the condition.

WHAT IS ACNE?

Acne is an inflammatory condition of the sebaceous glands, which explains its prevalence where these glands are most active: on the face, neck, back and chest. Excess sebum blocks the hair follicles and pores, allowing bacteria to build up and form the familiar spots and blemishes.

In a survey carried out by the medical press conducted amongst a group of schoolchildren, the majority believed that both diet and hormonal activity played a significant part in causing or aggravating acne.

Hormones cannot, of course, be manufactured without an adequate supply of correct nutrients in the diet. An excess of the wrong kinds of foods, particularly the wrong kinds of dietary fats, does seem to increase sebaceous gland activity. The usual teenage diet of chips, burgers, cola, sweets, chocolate and other junk foods is an open invitation to skin problems at a time when hormone activity is at its peak.

Other causes include poor elimination of toxic substances via a sluggish bowel, or a malfunctioning or congested liver, inadequate kidney function or poor expulsion of waste matter through the pores of the skin.

The relationship between skin disorders and the proper functioning of the large bowel is hardly ever discussed in medical circles but is a cornerstone of treatment in natural medicine. In my experience with case history studies, the majority of acne sufferers have chronic constipation or some other bowel or digestive disorder. Such will, of course, be aggravated by the persistent use of antibiotics!

COMEDOMES

Blackheads – or comedomes – are not, in fact, caused by dirt but by the oxidizing effect of air upon the sebum in a clogged pore and the skin's own colouring pigment called melanin. Comedomes penetrate deep into the skin but, with the right kind of skin care, can be removed. Facial saunas help to loosen the blockages and bring them to the surface. Steam which contains plant extracts such as chamomile, sage, echinacea and aloe vera can make this process even more effective. Face masks and scrubs will, with regular use, also encourage blackheads to the surface. Kaolin masks are particularly beneficial in treating blackheads and whiteheads (known as milia); the chalk in the mask is able to attract and absorb the oil in the blocked pore. Some authorities recommend a comedo extractor – a small metal tool which draws accumulated waste out of the pore or pimple. My own experience of these gadgets is that they are best left to the expert beautician and are not recommended for personal use. Unless guided gently and with dexterity, they can cause bruising and permanent harm.

A word of warning: However tempting it may be, NEVER squeeze blackheads. Apart from the risk of cross-infection, there is a strong likelihood that the pores will be so bruised and damaged that they will be unable to work properly ever again. Even touching the face can increase the number of spots and boils. Underneath the facial area there are lymph glands and sinus cavities. Surface inflammation caused by squeezing can result in far more serious (even fatal) infections if these areas are affected.

NOT JUST TEENAGERS

Of course, acne does affect other age groups too and pre-period flare-ups can be a common and unwelcome part of premenstrual syndrome. Dietary changes together with supplementation can relieve both the acne and the PMS.

Whilst acne vulgaris is most common during puberty, acne rosacea occurs chiefly in middle age. Common signs and symptoms are a flushed, red face sometimes accompanied by severe dryness and irritation around the chin, cheeks, nose and forehead. Extreme heat or cold – or sudden changes of temperature – are likely to aggravate the rosacea condition.

DIGESTION CONNECTION

The most likely cause of acne rosacea seems to be faulty digestion, possibly aggravated by certain suspect foods – particularly coffee, chocolate, oranges, orange juice, spices and alcohol, the latter causing swelling and acute redness of the nose.

Vitamins B_1 and B_2 are particularly helpful in the treatment of acne rosacea, for they are involved in protein metabolism and in feeding the nerves in the skin.

For surface treatment, I have found Bach Flower Rescue Cream to be very soothing and healing. Several interesting studies show that acne rosacea sufferers may also have hydrochloric acid and pancreatic enzyme deficiency. Following my list of recommendations on how to improve digestion should help. In addition, I would strongly suggest a consultation with a practitioner who specializes in treating digestive disorders and who is familiar with nutritional treatments. A few months of hydrochloric acid, pepsin and digestive enzyme supplementation can work wonders.

So don't give up hope! There is much that can be done to improve skin condition, reduce scarring and discourage flare-ups, simply by making healthful dietary changes, using tried and tested cleansing techniques and sensible supplements.

Certain foods seem to aggravate inflammation so, if acne or oily skin is a problem, try to avoid the following:

- [X] Red meat
- [X] Chocolate
- [X] Cow's milk
- [X] Sugar
- [X] Cola
- [X] Oranges
- [X] Wheat-based cereals
- [X] Alcohol
- [X] Processed, tinned and packeted food
- [X] Battery raised eggs or poultry
- [X] Deep fried and fatty foods
- [X] Cheese
- [X] Coffee
- [X] Sugary and carbonated drinks
- [X] Orange juice
- [X] Salt
- [X] Spicy food

Instead, choose:

- Any fresh fruit (except oranges and orange juices). Aim for two pieces of fruit every day, between meals or before meals but not with other food
- Fresh vegetables and salads. Include a salad and at least two fresh vegetables every day
- Home-made soups
- Wholegrains such as rice and rye, but avoid wheat-based products as much as possible

- Live bio-yoghurt (two or three small tubs each week) containing the friendly bacteria *Lactobacillus acidophilus* and *Bifido bacterium*
- Garlic, onions, leeks and shallots. Use them in salads, stews, soups and casseroles
- Seeds and nuts: sunflower, pumpkin and linseeds, brazils and almonds
- Fresh fish twice weekly
- Free-range poultry twice weekly
- Free-range eggs – three per week
- Filtered or bottled water. It is particularly important for acne and oily skin sufferers to drink plenty of fresh, clean fluids. Check out the chapter on internal detoxification (p.95) for more information
- Vegetable juices and diluted fruit juices
- One tablespoon of Lecithin granules daily, added to juices or breakfast cereals. Choose those which are rich in phosphatidyl choline

MORE ACNE AMMUNITION

Multiple deficiencies of certain nutrients are common in acne sufferers, usually due to a combination of poor diet, poor absorption and rapid growth. Frequently lacking are zinc, magnesium, selenium and chromium (see 'Skin Nutrients', p.55).

But not all supplements are beneficial; some can make matters much worse, especially if they are of poor quality or are not well absorbed. For example, both iron and iodine can be helpful in treating acne and yet I have found some supplements containing ferrous sulphate iron or too much iodine (such as kelp tablets) are best avoided. Taking large doses of multivitamins can also aggravate acne in some people; low doses are usually sufficient and, in my experience, more effective. A suitable multivitamin complex – containing the B complex vitamins, and vitamins A, C and E – should be adequate. Acne in men has shown some improvement following supplementation with a low dose of selenium (100–200mcg daily).

Vitamin A (as retinol) has also demonstrated exceptional improvements in both kinds of acne but, again, supplementation should be treated with respect and used under practitioner supervision. Where there is a shortage of vitamin A, boils, blackheads and whiteheads appear to be far more common. Vitamin A helps to speed healing, reduce soreness and regulate cell turnover.

The overactivity of the sebaceous glands which pump out excess sebum has been linked to a possible GLA deficiency. Regular supplements of evening primrose oil or Mega GLA can be of great benefit to acne and oily skin sufferers as they do seem to reduce inflammation and 'settle' those over-stimulated glands.

CARING FOR ACNE AND OILY SKIN ON THE OUTSIDE

It can be difficult to take in, but the fact is that one of the best cleansers for oily skin is oil. Water-based astringents may appear to do an effective job initially but the results are short-lived and, by their very nature, drying agents will encourage even greater production of sebum to compensate.

Proper skin care is vital and there are now some excellent and very effective products available. Regular use of cleansing lotions, scrubs to exfoliate dead skin cells, massage creams for gentle facial massage, face packs and moisturizers will all assist in improving skin texture and quality. Toning lotions are useful for freshening the skin and removing traces of cleanser but cold water splashes after cleansing seem to be just as effective. This 'action' causes a 'reaction' – the cold water attracting warm blood to the capillaries at the skin's surface, increasing circulation, improving the transport of healing nutrients and hastening the removal of waste. For very inflamed skin, you could try a facial wash made from an infusion of the herb Golden Seal; good health food shops should have Golden Seal loose or in tea bags.

Oily backs are also a common problem with acne sufferers. Use a back brush and mildly medicated body wash to gently exfoliate the skin and improve circulation.

Over the years, I have developed my own skin-care routine which, although it may not conform to the norm, has proved to be very effective in preventing eruptions, reducing oiliness, improving smoothness and enhancing general skin quality. You may like to try it out for yourself, adapting my suggestions to your own needs. The Resources section on p.218 may also be of assistance.

In the Morning

Cleanse
Use a pH-balanced cleanser (in bar or liquid form). Massage the cleanser into wet skin and rinse thoroughly with warm water. Complete all rinsing routines with a cold water splash.

Tone

To reduce the open appearance of enlarged pores, soak a cotton pad in a dilute mixture of cider vinegar and filtered water; one tablespoon of vinegar per cup of water. Any unused amount will keep in the fridge for two to three days. Toners do not actually close the pores but the action of bringing blood to the skin's surface plumps the skin and makes it 'tighten'.

Protect and Nourish

Use a protective day moisturizer and, if liked, an oil-free medicated foundation.

For Your Evening Routine

Cleanse

Choose a quality cold-pressed oil and massage a small amount well into the skin with clean fingers. Keep working the oil over the skin for two or three minutes. Next, remove any excess with a dry cotton pad, followed by further cotton pads wrung out in hand-hot water – or use a damp cosmetic sponge. (Don't use tissues for this job. Their wood-pulp base can scratch and irritate the delicate surface of the skin.)

Tone

Splash the face with cool water and dry with a clean towel.

Protect and Nourish

Choose a moisturizer suitable for oily or blemished skin and massage a small amount over the whole of the face. The eyes and neck areas also require special attention even if the skin is oily (see 'Beauty Tips' on pp.182 and 185).

Powders?

Avoid the use of compressed powder (the powder pad is a great way to cross-infect and increase spots) or loose powder (which can block the pores). A more effective option are tiny paper sheets (in miniature book form) which are impregnated with powder. There's no risk of spillage so no mess. They are hygienic, lightweight and fit easily into make-up purse, handbag or pocket. All you need to do is tear out a new page and blot the oily areas.

Scrubs

Exfoliating scrubs or peeling creams should be used two or three times per week (in the morning) after cleansing but before the cold water splash. This is a useful treatment for unclogging pores and removing accumulated debris. There are lots of excellent ready-made exfoliants available or you can make your own from kitchen ingredients such as oatbran or seasalt mixed to a 'paste' with water. Take care not to scrub too hard, especially over inflamed areas. Cosmetic sponges or flannel face cloths will help to remove surface skin cells too – but it is vital to use a new sponge or cloth for every application to avoid cross-infection. And do be gentle!

Steaming

Water vapour is very cleansing; regular steaming of oily, spotty skin dislodges dirt and bacteria, unclogs pores and improves circulation. First, remove all traces of make-up with a cleansing milk. Wipe away any excess but don't splash with cold water. Then, either lean over a basin of just boiled water for five minutes or use a facial sauna. Whilst the skin is still warm and damp, apply one of the following masks.

Face Packs

I have found some face packs – especially those recommended for oily skin – to be too drying. Nowadays, I produce my own pack, as and when I need it, in the kitchen with the following ingredients:

Three teaspoons of plain full-fat bio-yoghurt
One teaspoon of kaolin powder or Fuller's Earth
One teaspoon of oatmeal
or
One tablespoon of oatmeal
One lightly beaten free-range egg (small size)
One teaspoon fresh lemon juice

Mix together and spread over cleansed skin, avoiding the eye area. Cover the eyes with used tea bags, slices of cucumber skin or damp cotton pads soaked in herbal eyebright solution. Lie down quietly away from light and noise for 15 minutes and practise those deep breathing exercises explained in the chapter 'Breath of Life'. Rinse the pack with tepid water and then a cold water splash. Repeat once weekly.

Tea Tree Oil

Preparations containing Tea Tree Oil can be dabbed on to inflamed, spotty areas (use a clean cotton bud for each eruption to prevent cross-infection). Tea tree has natural antibiotic, antiseptic and antifungal properties and is also useful as a topical application for athlete's foot.

Whereas other antiseptics may damage tissue cells, tea tree oil can dissolve infection without harming the tissues. It sterilizes on contact and can prevent microbial growth for hours. It can be used for many different skin problems including burns, psoriasis, insect bites, herpes, even head lice! Do not, however, use tea tree oil internally. Whilst usually without side effects, it can cause sudden breathing difficulties and even anaphylactic shock (potentially fatal) in a few sensitive individuals; it can also cause reddening and irritation of the skin in some people. If you are in any doubt about your sensitivity to tea tree oil, use it diluted in extra virgin olive oil (one drop of tea tree to ten drops of olive oil).

PROBIOTICS

In my own practice, the use of *Lactobacillus acidophilus* and *Bifido bacterium* has demonstrated significant improvements in the treatment of skin disorders in general and acne and eczema in particular. For more information, refer to the chapter on skin nutrients, p.55.

CASE HISTORY

Marie came for her first consultation in February last year. She was 23 years old and getting married in July. She wanted to have 'one last shot' at trying to improve her skin condition before the wedding. One last shot because she felt she really had tried everything else.

Plagued by chronic acne vulgaris since the age of 13, it still covered her face, upper arms, back and shoulders. She had been given increasing doses of antibiotics and steroids over the previous 10 years, had seen four consultant dermatologists and had tried many creams and lotions. She was given the contraceptive pill by her G.P. but this had not helped either.

Sometimes, the condition would clear a little but always returned 'worse than before'. Her morale was low, she lacked confidence, was shy and reluctant to go out because she said she looked 'so awful'. School days had been miserable for her as she had suffered unpleasant teasing.

Other health problems included severe constipation, dull and oily hair, mouth ulcers, brittle nails covered in white flecks and a general lack of energy. When she first came to see me, her diet consisted mainly of convenience foods, 'T.V.' dinners, orange squash, white bread, red meat, coffee, tea, a few cooked vegetables and one or two pieces of fruit per week.

Her new diet included many changes and she began to enjoy a range of different foods including plenty of fresh fruit, a salad every day, oatmeal porridge, oat muesli, live yoghurt, fresh fish, vegetables, herbal teas and plenty of water to drink. She decreased her ordinary tea intake to two cups daily, giving up coffee altogether and drinking diluted apple and grape juice and vegetable juices instead. She also enjoyed organic cider vinegar and molasses mixed with hot boiled water as a warming winter drink.

She followed a course of herbal cleansing tablets, GLA, antioxidant vitamins A, C and E with a multi-mineral containing zinc and selenium. Her skin was completely clear in time for the wedding and has remained so. Her hair and nails are much improved, constipation is no longer a problem, she has not had any further mouth ulcers and her energy levels are, to use her own word, 'amazing'. She is thrilled with the recovery and feels much more confident and happy.

Eczema and Psoriasis

We've made great medical progress in the last generation. What used to be an itch is now an allergy.

Anonymous

Eczema
Psoriasis
Allergic Reactions
Food Testing
GLA
Evening Primrose Oil
Herbal Treatment
Digestion Connection
Bowel Toxicity
Treatment Checklist

ECZEMA

The word 'eczema' is derived from the Greek *ekzema* meaning to boil out or over. This simple explanation ties in neatly with the naturopathic view that the majority of skin diseases are external signs of internal disorder. The skin, being a major organ of elimination, is trying to bring the internal distress to the surface and 'boil it out'.

There are many different kinds of eczema which can strike any part of the body at any age. Red, inflamed, itchy and dry skin can erupt into a sore, blistering and oozing rash. Thickening, scaling skin is most likely to appear on the face, inner arms and legs - especially inside elbows and at the back of the knees.

No single, isolated cause has been found although food sensitivity, nutritional deficiency, the side effects of some drugs, absence of breast-feeding, stress and vaccinations have all been held responsible. In many cases, there is also a family history of eczema or associated conditions such as urticaria, asthma, hay fever, food intolerance or migraine. Asthma and eczema are common bedfellows.

Hydrocortisone creams and steroid drugs can give short-term relief but the condition will nearly always return when the medication ceases – and, of course, the side effects of these treatments need to be taken into consideration. The use of inhalers, commonly prescribed for the treatment of asthma and allergies, can also lead to the development of acne.

The complementary approach has shown much greater success, especially with regard to tracking down the food sensitivities which can aggravate the condition. Cow's milk, wheat products, tomatoes, potatoes, oranges, eggs, some kinds of fish, red meat, sugar, corn and some food colours and preservatives would appear to be the most common culprits, but any food can be a trigger and the level of reaction will vary between one individual and another. Removing the offenders from the diet – or eating them only occasionally in very small amounts – has reduced symptoms in many cases and given complete relief in others. But food exclusions should be regarded with caution. Eliminating too many items for too long a period (particularly from a child's diet) can do more harm than good and, in extreme circumstances, could cause severe malnourishment.

In my experience in practice, many 'allergies' can be related to poor digestion and inadequate absorption of nutrients. The skin often suffers an adverse reaction to a particular food simply because the body is unable to digest that food properly. Treating the digestive disorder first can result in an improvement in the skin condition but should be done only under the supervision of a qualified practitioner.

One of the safest ways of checking for sensitivity is to experiment by excluding certain food groups for seven to fourteen days at a time. This method of testing is useful not just for skin disorders but for a variety of other food-sensitive related conditions such as headaches and migraine. Once again, practitioner supervision is recommended since food testing is not only time-consuming but requires dedication and careful monitoring.

Favourite foods can be common miscreants and it may be difficult to avoid these without help and support. I have often heard patients exclaim surprise at the suggestion that a best-loved food may be causing them distress. 'This one definitely isn't a problem', they'll say. 'I eat it all the time.'

The following 'family' headings may be useful to anyone who would like to give food testing a try.

These tests are extensive and should be undertaken over a period of several months. By excluding only one complete group of foods for no more than two weeks, you should gain at least an insight into which food groups, if any, are likely to be aggravating your condition. Keep a diary of everything you eat and a note of if and when your condition worsens or improves. If a particular group is suspected, you can then move on to checking each individual food in that group to find out if it is the whole 'family' or just one 'member' which is causing distress.

You may not see complete resolution of the problem immediately – even if you isolate your sensitivity straight away – but, in the case of eczema, for example, you should have less irritation, reduced inflammation or redness and fewer new patches forming.

Never eliminate more than one group at a time and, if no suspects are found, reintroduce that group before eliminating the next one. The tests should not be followed by anyone who suffers from diabetes or any disorder that is receiving medical attention unless supervised by a G.P.

Food Families

Red Meat and Dairy Products
Butter; Cream; Beef and Beef products (including Hamburgers); All kinds of Liver; All kinds of Pâté; Gelatin and Gelatin products (including fruit jellies and capsule coatings on tablets); Lard; Beef Dripping; Cow's Milk and associated products made from Cow's Milk (including Cheese and Yoghurt); Goat's Milk and Goat's Yoghurt; Sheep's Yoghurt and Cheese made from Sheep's Milk; Lamb and Mutton; Pork and all Pork products (including Sausages, Pork Pies, Ham and Bacon); Venison and Veal.

Milk and beef are, of course, related products. Milk and meat extracts are used in a variety of convenience foods too, so check every label carefully, paying particular attention to stock cubes, tinned soups, packaged foods and shop-bought cakes.

Milk allergies and poor digestion of milk are very common problems made worse by the fact that, as we grow older, our ability to digest the milk sugar (lactose) diminishes. The production of hydrochloric acid in the stomach lessens with age and hampers not only the digestion of the milk protein but also the absorption of calcium. Milk can cause unpleasant feelings of nausea, bloatedness, stomach pains and flatulence and is one of the most common allergens connected with skin disorders. It is also notoriously mucus-forming and has been associated with catarrh, gastro-intestinal bleeding and bowel disorders.

Fish, Poultry and Eggs
Chicken; Turkey; Duck; Goose; Game; Rabbit; All Fish and Seafood products; All kinds of Eggs.

Fish can cause a severe allergy in some people. If you react badly to seafood, you will probably already know it. Eggs can also be the source of hidden allergies. If you are unable to take fish oil capsules, linseed oil capsules are an excellent alternative.

Fruit and Nuts
All Fresh Fruit; All Dried Fruit; All Nuts; Honey; All kinds and colours of Sugar (including Fructose); Syrup; All Alcoholic Beverages; Vinegar.

Pay particular attention to the labels on tins and packets as most convenience foods contain sweetening of some kind. Avoid all the foods listed above but make sure you include plenty of peas, beans, root vegetables, potatoes, brown rice, lentils and grains. Also include plenty of extra salad items during this test, to compensate for the lack of fruit.

If you are having packaged cereals for breakfast, avoid any which are pre-sweetened or which contain fruit and nuts. As well as this, you will have to give up all fruit juices during this period, including grape and apple juice.

Salicylates
Cucumber; Tomato; All Dried Fruit; Blackberries; Gooseberries; Raspberries; Loganberries; Strawberries; Grape Juice; All Alcoholic Beverages; Vinegar; Almonds; Apples; Apricots; Plums; Prunes; Nectarines; Oranges; Satsumas; Clementines; Potatoes; Banana; Coffee (instant and ground); Pineapple; Liquorice.

Choosing what to eat instead may be a little more difficult during the term of this Salicylates test. Just avoid anything in the list or products which may contain any of the above items.

Salicylates are a group of foods which contain salicylic acid, a natural form of aspirin which can cause uncomfortable reactions in some people. During this trial, you should also avoid all proprietary medicines which contain aspirin. If, however, you are taking a prescribed tablet or medicine which you think may contain aspirin, check with your doctor first.

Grains and Grain Products
All Wheat and Wheat products (including pizzas; sauces made with flour, gravy thickening; bread, cakes, pastries – shop bought or home made); Pasta and Pasta products; Semolina; Rye; Barley; Millet; Maize (Corn) and associated products (Cornflour and Sweetcorn); Popcorn; Oats; All kinds of Rice; All kinds of Sugar including Raw Sugar, Brown Sugar, Molasses, Syrup and Treacle; grain-based drinks such as Beer and Whisky; All Yeast and Yeast products.

Whilst avoiding grain foods, eat plenty of fruit, yoghurt, eggs, cheese, jacket potatoes, meat, fish and salads.

Wheat is a common allergen which can cause or aggravate a range of bowel and digestive disorders

Vegetables – Section 1
(Test only one vegetable section at a time)

Cucumber; Courgettes; Marrow; Pumpkin and Pumpkin Seeds; Melon; All Dried Beans; All Sprouted Beans; Beansprouts; String and Runner Beans; Broad Beans; Peas; Potato; Red, Green and Yellow Peppers; Pimento; Chilli; Paprika; Cayenne; Fenugreek; Carob and Carob Chocolate; Soya and associated items (including Soya Oil, Soya Milk and Soya Lecithin); Tofu; Sesame Seeds, Sesame Oil and Sesame Butter (Tahini); Linseed; Tobacco.

For lunch and for your evening meal, choose fish, meat, bread, brown rice and fruit. Salad and vegetables are acceptable as long as they do not include items in the above list.

Tomato, tobacco, potato, pimento, peppers, paprika, aubergine, chilli and cayenne all belong to the Deadly Nightshade family and can cause unpleasant reactions in some people due to the natural chemical solanine.

Vegetables – Section 2 (including Herbs and Spices)
All these herbs and spices: Angelica; Aniseed; Basil; Bay; Bergamot; Cardomon; Caraway; Chervil; Coriander; Cinnamon; Cumin; Dill; Fennel; Ginger; Marjoram; Oregano; Mace; Mint; Parsley; Peppermint and Spearmint; Nutmeg; White and Black Pepper; Poppy Seeds; Rosemary; Sage; Savory; Thyme; Tumeric; Vanilla; Garlic and all related Onion family foods including Leeks, Chives, Shallots and Spring Onions.

And these foods: Avocado; Asparagus; Bamboo Shoots; Beetroot; Carrot; Celeriac; Celery; Swiss Chard; Olives and Olive Oil; Parsnip; Sweet Potato; Tapioca; Yam and Chinese Water Chestnuts.

If you normally use Olive Oil, use Sesame Seed Oil instead during this test. Do beware of items such as Bouquet Garni, Stock Cubes and Flavourings which may contain several of the above items. Earl Grey tea is made from Bergamot leaves.

Vegetables - Section 3
Brussels Sprouts; Broccoli; Burdock; Cauliflower; Chamomile; Chicory; Chinese Leaves; Dandelion; Globe and Jerusalem Artichoke; Endive; Horseradish; Kale; Kohlrabi; Lettuce; Mustard; Mustard and Cress; Salsify; Sunflower Seeds and Sunflower Oil (including your margarine if it contains sunflower oil); Tarragon; Turnips and Turnip Greens; Watercress.

Caffeine
Coffee (instant, ground and decaffeinated); Ceylon, China and Indian Teas; All Cola drinks; Chocolate and all products containing chocolate; Cocoa and Drinking Chocolate.

Coffee and tea are often the most difficult items to give up even for a short space of time. Take things easy and don't make your life miserable by doing entirely without - if you really feel you can't. Extend this particular test over three or four weeks if you like. You are not being forced to give up tea and coffee on a permanent basis - only to discover if you have any unpleasant reactions to them which may be affecting your health and well-being. It is also worth experimenting with different kinds of coffee and tea. I know patients who react badly to one brand but not to another. Generally, the more expensive, quality brands contain less caffeine – and taste better too (see Resources p.218).

Evening Primrose Oil and Herbal Medicine

In recent years, there have also been major steps forward in the treatment of eczema using natural medicine. The first was the discovery of a problem common to eczema sufferers – that they have low levels of essential fatty acid metabolites, suggesting an inability to convert these vital nutrients into usable form. There may also be a straightforward dietary deficiency of EFAs. Giving GLA (gamma linolenic acid) supplements appears to bypass this 'block' in the metabolic pathway and an increasing number of studies have now been carried out which demonstrate the beneficial action of GLA in the relief of itching and inflammation. One result of this work is that evening primrose oil (its active ingredient is GLA) is now available on prescription for eczema.

Although Western medics are slow to accept the astonishing results, another breakthrough has been the discovery that Chinese herbal medicine may be able to provide the all-clear for an eczema cure. Inspired by a herbalist based in London's Soho who has an 85 per cent success rate in clearing eczema using individual treatments, a study was set up at Great Ormond Street Children's Hospital in London in 1991. More than 60 per cent of the patients taking part in this trial showed a significant improvement in their skin condition. Unfortunately, there have been a small number of reported cases of liver toxicity in a few ultra-sensitive individuals. It may therefore be prudent to undergo liver and kidney function tests prior to commencement of treatment.

PSORIASIS

This is a skin disease of many varieties characterized by scaly circular or ring-shaped patches of thickened, red and dry skin, most common on the elbows, knees, legs and torso. Some experts will tell you that itching is rare in psoriasis sufferers, but my experience with new patients would suggest that the irritation and desire to scratch are often the most distressing symptoms.

In psoriasis, skin cells reproduce many hundreds of times more quickly than normal, causing constant flaking and scaling of the affected areas.

Unknown Causes

The cause remains unknown but excessive stress, poor eating habits, liver and kidney malfunction, bacterial and viral infections, chronic irritation, burns, poor elimination, food intolerances, essential fatty acid deficiencies, multiple nutrient deficiencies including zinc and vitamin A and a gunked-up colon have all been implicated in causing or aggravating the condition. So too have prescribed drugs such as lithium carbonate (for manic and psychotic disorders), anti-hypertensives (for high blood pressure), anti-malarial drugs, NSAIDs (the non-steroidal anti-inflammatory drugs used in arthritis), and the sudden withdrawal of steroid drugs.

Orthodox Treatment

The powerful drugs, creams and coal tar preparations available may help to relieve some symptoms but cannot bring about a cure. Indeed, the side effects of these items can be more bothersome than the condition they are meant to treat.

Whereas eczema has a contiguous link with asthma, psoriasis and arthritis have a close association with each other; both conditions affecting the same person or there being a connection through family history. It is common to find sufferers saddled with a complicated regime of drugs which may be aggravating rather than alleviating the symptoms.

The Food Family testing outlined above is more commonly used in cases of eczema, but it would certainly be worth a try in the treatment of psoriasis. Gluten allergy has also been discovered in a number of psoriasis sufferers.

Improving diet quality by increasing intake of fresh oily fish and taking fish oil capsules, but *avoiding* citrus fruits, nuts, corn, milk, coffee and tomatoes has been shown to benefit psoriasis sufferers; while treating digestive disorders, making time for rest and relaxation, taking Omega 3 and Omega 6 EFA supplements, eradicating constipation, improving bowel, liver and spleen function, taking probiotics to repopulate the friendly flora and undergoing colonic irrigation have demonstrated startling results in a range of skin disorders.

Poor Digestion

The link between skin disorders and food intolerance has often incriminated the 'leaky gut' as a co-factor in the progression of the disease. 'Gut leakiness' means what it says. When foods are broken down inadequately, partially digested substances irritate the gastro-intestinal lining, causing inflammation. As a result of these localized swellings the gut wall becomes increasingly permeable, allowing larger than usual particles of food to find their way through into the bloodstream.

Unfortunately, these bits of food are not welcome here. The immune system - which hasn't been told about the stomach inflammation and the extra-large gaps in the gut wall - sees these particles as invaders. The result is an allergic response. The anti-invader alarm system is sounded and the body systems are alerted to the allergen. Symptoms may include increased digestive discomfort, breathing difficulties, skin irritation and loose bowel movements.

Treating the underlying digestive malfunction and taking specialized supplements designed to heal a 'holey' gut may be enough, in many cases, to fix the leak and settle the skin condition at the same time. Production of the protective fatty acid called butyric acid, formed during the colonic fermentation of dietary fibre, is reduced where a leaky gut condition exists. Butyrates are believed to reduce the risk of bowel cancer. Butyric acid supplements are available but are generally only available from practitioners.

Another condition which can cause a leaky gut is candidiasis, a yeast imbalance which can be treated through dietary changes and the consumption of probiotics (see pp.40 and 77, and Resources).

Bowel Toxicity

According to the American naturopath Dr Bernard Jensen, autointoxication of the blood and tissues together with a silted, impacted colon are major factors in the aetiology of skin disease. The cell proliferation associated with psoriasis is increased markedly where unfriendly bacteria have overflowed and penetrated the gut wall. Colonic irrigation, associated with cleansing foods and probiotic supplements, has shown remarkable results in the treatment of psoriasis. Dr Jensen's book *Tissue Cleansing Through Bowel Management* is particularly instructive in this regard – but is definitely not for the squeamish! You'll need a strong stomach to study the colour photographs which show the colon debris taken from some chronic psoriasis sufferers.

ECZEMA AND PSORIASIS – TREATMENT CHECKLIST

- Avoid wearing rough-textured or wool clothing next to the skin. Wear natural cotton fibres. Thermal fabrics and mohair can be particularly irritating.
- Choose washing suds and fabric softeners that are designed specifically for sensitive skin.
- Bathe and shower in warm water – never very hot or very cold.
- Never use ordinary soap. It's too alkaline and drying.
- Avoid sudden changes of temperature wherever possible.
- Moderate and sensible exposure to sunlight and fresh air can be most beneficial so try to spend time out of doors.
- Reduce irritation with hypericum and calendula homoeopathic cream, vitamin E cream, Derma-C or Golden Seal lotion.
- Check your stress levels. Can you do anything to reduce them? Relaxation therapy, aromatherapy, reflexology, tai chi and yoga can all be helpful in 'teaching' the body how to cope with excessive and negative stress.
- Even if you can't track down any food sensitivities, check the quality of your diet. Are you eating enough fresh fruits, vegetables, salads, seeds, nuts and wholegrains? Perhaps there

are a few too many chocolate bars, ready meals or take-aways?

- Ask to be referred to an experienced herbalist and/or nutrition practitioner so that your diet can be investigated and any possible food intolerances tested.

These supplements have all demonstrated their usefulness in treating a wide variety of skin conditions:

- Evening primrose oil or GLA. Evening primrose oil is available on prescription in the U.K. for eczema
- Fish oil or linseed oil supplements – anti-inflammatory
- Vitamin A – fights infection and reduces dryness; 10,000 iu daily
- Vitamin C – a multi-functional skin nutrient; 2 grams daily
- Bioflavonoids – balances histamine production (follow pack dosage instructions)
- Vitamin E – essential for renewal of healthy cells; 400–600 iu daily
- Probiotics – restores natural balance of gut ecology (usually one or two capsules daily)
- Sarsaparilla – helps to bind bacterial toxins (follow pack dosage instructions)
- Selenium (antioxidant) – 100–200 mcg daily
- Silymarin – a liver-cleansing herb (follow pack dosage instructions)
- Zinc citrate (helps healing) – 15–25 mg per day

For details of further reading and skin disorder clinics, see pp.214 and 218.

Hair Essentials

This is that Lady of Beauty, in whose praise
Thy voice and hand shake still – long known to thee
By flying hair and fluttering hem . . .

From 'Soul's Beauty' by Dante Gabriel Rossetti (1828–82)

> Hair and Scalp Health
> Split Ends
> Scalp Massage
> Cleansing Diets
> Hormone Levels
> Medication
> Hair-Care Plan
> Hair Loss

Hair condition is very sensitive to alterations in atmosphere, environment and lifestyle; any changes in our health and well-being will usually show quickly in the hair. Our 'crowning glory' is not fundamental to survival and so will be the first to lose its supply of nutrients in any crisis. Consequently, hair may appear lacklustre and lifeless, dry and brittle or lank and oily at the earliest sign of stress or illness.

Hair is not just there for decoration or embellishment. It acts to protect the skull and the brain from physical damage, as a screen from the sun's rays, as a valuable sensor (you always notice immediately when someone or something brushes even lightly against your hair) and it keeps the head warm.

The health of the scalp and quality of the hair which grows from it are largely determined by the level of nutrients supplied to the body and how effective the bloodstream is at carrying them to where they are needed.

Each scalp has an average of 100,000 hairs, although blondes usually have more - around 120,000 - and redheads less - 80,000 or so. A natural hair fall in the region of 100 hairs each day is perfectly normal, although shedding will occur in greater or lesser amounts at different times of the year.

Each strand of hair is made up of dead protein cells (keratin) constructed in overlapping layers. When the layers lie flat and smooth, each hair reflects the light, making it shine. When the strata are peeling or raised, no light is reflected and hair appears dull and lifeless. Unloved hair exposed to too much sun, perming, bleaching, tinting, central heating, curling tongs and blow drying at too high a temperature is likely to be dry, dull and brittle. Split ends may travel right up the hair shaft if not trimmed regularly.

Tension in the scalp and neck - with its consequent detriment to blood supply and circulation of nutrients - is often alone responsible for hair and scalp disorders. Massaging the scalp before hair-washing, as outlined in the Hair Care Plan below, can be enormously beneficial.

And if you have ever wondered why hair 'stands on end' when you are nervous or frightened, this is the remains of a reaction designed to make you look taller and terrify your enemy!

GETTING THE BALANCE RIGHT

Hair has its own inbuilt moisturizer called sebum - the oily substance produced by the sebaceous glands. When hair suffers from dryness, the cause can be often related to lack of sebum production or, alternatively, to the inability of the natural oil to reach all the hair. In long hair or in tight curls, for example, or where hair is damaged, sebum has more difficulty travelling along the hair shaft.

As soon as hair is washed, the sebum coating is lost. But hair left unwashed can create both hygiene and health difficulties; so we overcome the problem by using conditioners.

Dull, oily hair may be the result of poor elimination of wastes and toxins, poor circulation, inadequate fluid intake, a sluggish bowel – or of being simply 'below par'. In these circumstances, a regular cleansing diet with herbal and vitamin supplements may be called for.

HAIR AND HORMONES

The contraceptive pill, which alters hormone levels in the body, may trigger a thinning of hair in some people. Temporary, sudden hair loss – caused by a reduction in oestrogen levels – can occur in a mother who has just given birth. The hair will grow back but both of these situations should be helped considerably by the introduction of a multivitamin/mineral supplement and the addition of essential fatty acids to the diet.

MEDICATION

Many drug medicines – as well as anaesthetics – are known to have a detrimental effect upon hair condition, causing hair loss in some people. Also, a sudden whitening of hair can occur following illness or drug therapy. No-one should stop taking their prescribed medication without first seeking their doctor's advice, but some dietary changes and well-chosen supplements can make a significant difference to hair and scalp condition in such circumstances.

CONDITION IS EVERYTHING

Whether you are blessed with straight, curly, frizzy, thick or thin hair is determined by your genes. But for those of us who are not satisfied with the type of hair Nature bestowed upon

Hair condition can be affected by many other things too:

Too much sun	Drying wind
Overexposure to salt air	Stress
Chlorinated water	Illness
Nervous disorders	Inadequate rest and relaxation
Lack of exercise	Shallow breathing
Crash dieting	Thyroid insufficiency
X-ray treatments	Chemotherapy
Shock	Trauma

Scalp condition may suffer as a result of:

Seborrhoeic Dermatitis	Eczema
Psoriasis	Acne
Dandruff	

Hair and scalp can also be detrimentally affected by:

Pollution	Poor-quality diet
Nutrient deficiency	

us, it is important to know how to keep treated hair in good condition. Straightening curly hair, perming straight locks into corkscrew kinks, colouring the grey or bleaching in the highlights can all inflict untold damage.

HAIR CARE PLAN

- Wash hair more frequently. Leaving it for too long between washes can make it more brittle and lifeless because dead skin cells and impurities are allowed to build up.
- Massage the scalp before every wash. This will loosen those dead cells, improve circulation and encourage growth. And contrary to myth, it's good for greasy hair. Scalp massage is also a great stress reliever. Place a thumb behind each ear and spread out the fingers. Press gently on to the scalp and, with the finger tips (not the nails), move the skin of the scalp over the bones of the skull. Work from the back of the neck, upwards and over the top of the head to the brow. Never tear at the hair or rub it vigorously.
- Wet the hair thoroughly before shampooing. Use a gentle shampoo and a conditioner at each wash. It isn't necessary to shampoo twice; one application is sufficient. Shampoos that create lots of lather are not necessarily the best kind; the more foam, the harsher the shampoos may be.
- Try to use a 'matching set' of products but don't stick to that same make all the time. Find three or four brands that you like and alternate between them. Choose those which contain vitamins and plant extracts and which haven't been tested on animals.
- Rinse hair really thoroughly after shampooing – both before and after applying conditioner. Never use water that is too hot. Warm water is best followed by a cool final rinse.

- Don't rub too briskly. Treat hair with extra respect when it is wet. Blot dry and comb through using a wide-toothed comb GENTLY.
- When possible, allow hair to dry naturally.
- Every two weeks use a special cleansing shampoo to remove the build-up of gels, mousses and conditioners.
- Keep hair dryer settings low. Damage is not done by drying but by *over*-drying and excessive heat whether from blow-dryers, curling wands or heated rollers.
- Once each day, brush the hair from the nape of the neck towards the forehead and, if possible, bend forwards at the same time so that the blood – literally – rushes to the head. Take care, however; this procedure is helpful to hair but can cause light-headedness. Gentle exercise – and, if you are agile enough and do not have heart or blood pressure problems, head and shoulder stands – are beneficial.
- Don't over-brush the hair. The old wives' tale about 100 strokes per night is just that – an old wives' tale. Such action makes the hair greasy and can do lots of damage! It was recommended for spreading sebum along the hair shaft in the days before conditioners.
- Hair can become very brittle and 'flyaway' in cold weather. Central heating and air conditioning don't help either. Add condition and reduce static by using a little hair wax when combing through.
- Hot oil treatments are useful for deep conditioning. Or you can use oils such as olive, apricot or almond from the kitchen cupboard. Pour about a tablespoon of oil into an egg cup or small bowl and stand the container in a larger dish of hot water. When the oil is warm, massage it gently into the hair. Split open a polythene bag and wrap it over the hair, keeping it in place with a warm towel. Curl up in a cosy corner for 15 to 30 minutes and relax. Then remove

the towel and the polythene wrap. Work a good 'dollop' of shampoo into the hair (before wetting it). Then rinse. Shampoo a second time, rinse again, apply your usual conditioner and then give a final and thorough rinse.

- Grapeseed oil makes a wonderful conditioner. Two tiny drops rubbed between the palms and then through damp hair works well for all hair types.
- To revitalize lacklustre hair or an itchy scalp, pierce open a couple of vitamin E capsules and massage the contents into the roots. Comb gently and leave oil in place for several hours, preferably overnight.
- Aloe vera juice is an excellent revitalizer for tired and dull hair. Its chemical composition is very similar to that of keratin so it is able to penetrate the hair shaft. A few spoonfuls of juice poured over the hair after the final rinse will nourish, protect and shine.
- Nettle tea makes an excellent hair rinse and is a useful treatment for dandruff.
- Many herbs are excellent hair helpers due to their natural anti-bacterial and anti-fungal properties. Chamomile improves hair's shine because it contains natural polymers which add shine to each strand. Calendula, clove, hops, juniper, rosemary, sage, thyme and yarrow help to control dandruff. Oiliness can be curtailed with wild-cherry bark, red clover or horsetail (which is rich in the trace mineral silica). Horsetail is also believed to be a hair strengthener, reducing the risk of split ends and breakage. Many of these herbs are now finding their way into hair products.
- Keep all combs and brushes scrupulously clean.
- Use natural bristle brushes and wide-toothed combs – they are more gentle on the hair.
- Even if you are trying to grow your hair, have the ends trimmed every eight weeks or so.

- Always use both shampoo and conditioner after swimming. Simple rinsing without shampoo is not enough to remove either salt or chlorine.
- Hairspray landing on the face can cause spots; ask your hairdresser about a plastic face guard to hold in front of the face while spraying.

GOOD FOODS FOR HAIR HEALTH

Live yoghurt, fresh oily fish, fresh vegetables and salads, fresh fruits, cold-pressed oils (but don't cook with them), sunflower seeds, pumpkin seeds, sesame seeds, linseeds, pulses, sea vegetables, wholegrains such as brown rice and oats, buckwheat, millet, almonds, fresh fish, lecithin granules, figs and dates – and plenty of filtered water.

TRY TO AVOID THESE HAIR HINDERERS

Too much cow's milk or cheese can be detrimental to hair condition, as can diets high in caffeine, cola, chocolate, sugar, salt, saturated and hydrogenated fats, food additives and nicotine.

SUPPLEMENTS FOR HEALTHY HAIR

All the B vitamins – particularly B_3, B_5, choline, inositol and para-amino benzoic acid. Some researchers say that PABA is helpful in reducing the likelihood of premature greying; however, it is unlikely to make any significant difference to hair that has already turned grey. Gamma linolenic acid (GLA), fish oil and linseed oil are all beneficial to hair, scalp and skin. The antioxidant nutrients – vitamins A, C, E, selenium and zinc – should be included in any supplement programme for the hair.

LOSING YOUR LOCKS?

Thinning hair can sometimes be related to poor digestion of proteins, so that improving digestion and absorption will often result in new and thicker growth (see 'The Importance of Good Digestion', p.89).

Common hair loss (alopecia) is a rather different problem which is hormone-related and which affects 50 to 60 per cent of men (male-pattern baldness) and 10 per cent of women.

Man has been obsessed with hair loss and baldness down the ages. Myriad lotions, potions, pills and contraptions have been invented and discarded in the quest for hair re-growth. But despite fervent and ongoing investigations, nothing would persuade falling locks to stop falling.

In recent years, a specialist treatment for serious hair disorders has been developed by Italian doctors. The results of their extensive research and the clinical trials carried out worldwide have been impressive. Although not a hair restorer or cure for baldness, this non-drug therapy has shown good results in reducing hair loss, encouraging re-growth and thickening of hair and helping seborrhoeic dermatitis. For further information see Resources.

Nails and Hands

Do you suffer with problem nails which break or split well before they ever reach a decent length? Don't give up - it's easy to grow them longer, stronger and shinier.

Nail condition, like that of hair and skin, can mirror your health. But apart from lacking nourishment, nails will also suffer if they are overexposed to very hot water, detergents, central heating, air conditioning, cold biting winds, too much tap-tapping away at the keyboard or overuse of stick-on nails.

A report from the *British Journal of Dermatology* suggests that putting hands directly into washing suds and other detergents may cause skin rashes, soreness and irritation even at low concentrations. The study showed that people who were not normally allergic suffered itching and redness when their skin was in contact with only a mild solution of washing up liquid. Exposure was only of short duration - 15 minutes three times a day for three weeks. Volunteers who wore household gloves or used only warm tap water were not affected. So always use rubber gloves for washing up and/or a protective barrier cream too.

WHAT ARE NAILS THERE FOR?

Nails are the evolutionary remains of claws. They protect the ends of the fingers from damage, enhance our sensitivity to touch and enable us to pick up, handle and manipulate the smallest of objects.

The delicate fold of skin at the base of the nail is called the cuticle. The hard part which grows out from the 'half moon' is called the nail plate, a hard protein substance very similar in structure to that of the hair.

The cells in the nail plate are no longer living cells – which is why we don't experience pain when the nail tips are filed, cut or damaged. However, the area just under the 'half moon' or lunula is composed of active cells which, when healthy, are constantly renewing the plate and pushing it forward.

FIX FRAIL NAILS

Good circulation and a constant supply of nutrients help to give the nail structure its strength, pliability and resistance to damage. Caring for nails internally and externally is really worth the effort but it takes time to achieve results. Fingernails grow slowly – at a rate of about 1mm each week. Where health is under par or there is a deficiency of the right kind of nutrients, growth may be very slow indeed. Conversely, excessive stress (including nail biting or cuticle nibbling!) may over activate new cell production, causing the nail to grow too quickly. On average, it takes three to four months for a nail to renew itself from base to tip and about six or seven months to replenish completely. So poor-quality nails may be reflecting your previous state of health too.

NAIL NUTRIENTS

White flecks on the nails may indicate zinc deficiency but supplementing with individual zinc tablets is not always the most sensible answer. Your diet may already contain enough zinc which is, perhaps, poorly absorbed – or you may be short of other nutrients such as manganese, copper or B vitamins which help zinc to work. Isolated nutrients taken indiscriminately can cause imbalances of other nutrients so that it is possible to make matters even worse. If you really are low in zinc, better to have a 3-month course of a good-quality multivitamin/mineral complex which contains zinc than to take the zinc on its own. Before supplementing, check the list of symptoms in the 'Skin Nutrients' chapter, p.55, and see if you recognize any other indicators of zinc shortage. White marks may also be caused by the contraceptive pill or by minuscule air bubbles under the plate which are formed when the nail is knocked or the matrix (the part underneath and behind the half moon) or cuticle damaged.

Weak, pale or spoon-shaped nails may be the result of low iron reserves. However, the same rules apply as to zinc. Don't take separate iron supplements. Increase your intake of iron-rich foods (and vitamin C which helps iron absorption) and see your doctor if you suspect other iron-deficiency symptoms. Cut down your tea intake to a maximum of three cups a day. Too much tea robs the body of iron.

Delicate, fragile and ridged nails can also be due to lack of protein, vitamin A or calcium (see 'Skin Nutrients' p.55 for more information).

Swiss scientists have found that biotin, a member of the B group of vitamins, can strengthen poor-quality nails. Dramatic improvements were noted in 22 people with thin, brittle fingernails after a nine-month course of biotin at 2.5mg per day. Following treatment, splitting had partially or completely stopped; nails were also thicker and smoother.

One of the best nail nutrients I have found is GLA. Patients who have taken evening primrose oil or GLA supplements for another condition (for example pre-menstrual syndrome, breast pain or eczema) have often reported improved nail quality – as well as warmer extremities. Because GLA improves blood flow, it helps the circulation to the hands and feet – and nails! Recommended dosage is six 500mg capsules of evening primrose oil or an equivalent GLA product daily for six months. Remember that these nutrients can take many weeks to make a difference – so do persevere.

SUPER NAIL TIPS

- Witch hazel mixed 50:50 with cucumber juice is an excellent remedy for chapped hands. Rub the mixture in and leave it to dry.
- Fresh lemon juice massaged around the cuticles and under the nails will lift away ingrained dirt. Or try a tablespoon of olive oil with a tablespoon of brown sugar or sea salt.
- If you are ultra-sensitive to ordinary soaps and detergents, keep a bowl of oatmeal near the tap. It makes a great soap substitute. Wet the skin, rub the hands and nails thoroughly with the oatmeal and rinse with warm water. Or use non-alkaline glycerine and vegetable-oil based soaps.
- Help cracked or split cuticles by massaging them with Bach Flower Rescue Cream or Calendula and Hypericum Cream.

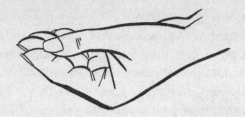

NOURISHING NAILS AND HANDS

All the information given here for fingernails applies to
toenails too.

Step One

Use a rich hand cream every night and a lighter hand lotion
during the day - especially after hands have been in water.
Work the cream thoroughly into the skin and be sure to
include the backs of the hands, knuckles, fingers and thumbs -
and the nails, pushing the cuticles gently back from the nail
as you go. Take great care not to tear at, jab or cut the skin
around the nails; this could disturb nail growth and thicken
the cuticle. Massaging in this way speeds the circulation and
improves the flow of nutrients, thereby encouraging new nail
growth. Wiggle and stretch the fingers for a few seconds at
regular intervals throughout the day to improve circulation and
release tension.

Step Two

Once or twice a week, soak your fingertips in a bowl of
warmed olive oil for five or ten minutes. For nails which are
in very poor condition, it helps to do this just before bedtime
and to put on a pair of cotton gloves after treatment so that
the oil can continue to work during the night.

Step Three

Use a fine-grain, professional-quality emery board for filing. I find the black or dark grey ones longer lasting, more effective and gentler than the two-tone kind (which look and feel like coarse sandpaper). Never use metal files – they tear the nail. Sawing backwards and forwards does the same, so always file in one direction only – from the sides to the centre. Aim for a neat oval shape and avoid sharp sides or points. Neat, short nails will be stronger than long ones. Filing can be done with old polish in place (it helps to strengthen and protect) but do remove it before conditioning or buffing. Clip or cut toenails straight across and finish off with gentle filing and buffing.

Step Four

A regular weekly buffing helps to smooth out ridges and improve blood flow. Take off old varnish with an acetone-free remover using a cotton pad or make-up remover disc. Apply a tiny amount of nail buffing paste (available from most chemists and drug stores) over each nail and rub it in with the opposing fingertip; or use a file-shaped polisher/buffer. Then, with long sweeping strokes, polish up with a buffer pad or piece of towelling cloth until you have achieved a natural shine. Rinse the hands with cool water, dry thoroughly and buff again. The shine will deepen with regular treatment.

Step Five

Protect with polish; it helps to give extra resilience. But avoid all varnishes until nail strength and quality have improved. Varnish removers (even gentle ones) can be very drying and may make matters worse if nails are 'under par'.

Before applying polish, remember to rinse any oil or cream from the nails.

For a perfect finish, use a base coat, followed by one or two layers of top colour. Allow 10–15 minutes between coats. And leave a little gap around the cuticle; painting right up to the skin prevents evaporation and can cause nails to soften.

Yellowing of the nails is most often caused by the use of very dark-coloured polish which stains if applied directly to the nail. Overcome the problem by avoiding deep-coloured varnish or make sure that you always use a protective base coat. Painting unvarnished nails several times a day with neat fresh lemon juice will bleach out any previous staining. Discolouration may also be due to smoking.

Hangnails are torn areas of skin at the side or base of a nail. They are common where skin is very dry, allowing cuticles to crack and split easily. Stress is also a factor since nibbling and chewing at the skin around the nails encourages hangnails. Good treatments are relaxation and deep breathing exercises, use of hand lotion after every wash and regular soaking of the fingers in warm olive oil. Hangnails which won't heal may indicate deficiencies of vitamin C or the B complex. Never trim or cut the cuticles; hangnails will repair given time and proper care.

Super Beauty Tips

She walks in beauty, like the night
  Of cloudless climes and starry skies;
And all that's best of dark and bright
  Meet in her aspect and her eyes . . .
                    Lord Byron (1788–1824), *Hebrew Melodies: She Walks in Beauty*

> The Face
> The Neck
> Make-up Kits
> Massage
> VDU Screens
> Eyes Right
> Lip Service
> On Your Toes

FACIAL FEAST

Salon facials can be a wonderful experience but can also be expensive. So why not give yourself a real treat at home?
Tie the hair back from the face. Rinse the face and neck with warm water. Remove excess but don't dry too thoroughly. Then apply your usual cleanser, massaging it gently for two or three minutes. Pour just-boiled water into a large bowl (fill the bowl in situ from the kettle; don't try carrying the bowl after it has been filled). Alternatively, use a facial sauna. Steam the skin for one minute (two minutes if the skin is oily). Next, wipe the face with damp cotton pads to remove remaining cleanser and impurities. Then return to the steam for a further minute (two or three for oily skin). After this, apply a face mask suited to your skin type.

For normal or dry skin, try avocado and banana mashed with a teaspoon of yoghurt. For oily skin, beat a small free-range egg with a teaspoon of lemon juice and a tablespoon of oatmeal – or try the packs described in the chapter on 'Acne', p.136.

Place cool cucumber slices or cold chamomile teabags over your eyes. Lie down in a darkened room away from noise and interruptions for 10 to 15 minutes.

Rinse the mask away with tepid water. Apply a scrub mixture of wet oatmeal and work it over the whole of the face and neck for a minute or so. Rinse again and follow with a cold splash or your favourite toner. Complete the treatment by applying your regular moisturizer and massaging it thoroughly into the face and neck.

MAKE-UP KITS

For tip-top skin health, it is important to care for your make-up equipment and applicators as carefully as you would look after your skin, or they can become happy breeding grounds for germs. It's best to use a jar to wash brushes, rather than a bowl or basin, so that you can keep handles out of the water (wooden handles will spoil and rot if you get them wet). Never leave brushes to soak: bristles will loosen and fall out. Allow equipment to dry naturally in a warm place, but away from direct heat. If brushes are stiff when dried, try shaking out excess water more vigorously next time; or rinse them in a drop of diluted fabric softener. Before washing brushes and combs, remove any loose hair and then agitate them in warm water and a squeeze of mild shampoo. Rinse with cool water and a dash of sterilizing fluid.

Never share your make-up or hair equipment with anyone. If you get an infection such as herpes, throw your applicators away and start again when the infection has gone.

NECKS AREN'T FUSSY – THEY'RE JUST THIRSTY

One of the easiest ways to determine age is by looking at the neck. The skin here has far fewer sebaceous glands than the face, making it more susceptible to dryness and premature ageing. The bust area (the body's natural bra) has no supportive muscle tissue and relies on the elasticity of the skin for support and shape. Test this out for yourself by placing your fingers inside the shoulders below the collar bone and pulling gently upwards. See how the breasts are lifted.

Many women spend several hours a week – and lots of hard-earned money – on caring for the face whilst ignoring the area between the chin and the bustline. I was always taught that the face ends where the bra begins! In other words, care for your neck and décolletage just as you would your face. Cleanse it, tone it, use your scrub and mask regularly, massage it – and, most important of all, moisturize, moisturize, moisturize!

A five-minute massage with moisturizer at the end of every day really is worth the effort. There are lots of special neck creams on the market but any good skin cream will do. The important thing is to apply that moisture to cleansed, exfoliated skin and massage it well into the whole neck area, shoulders, back of the neck, up to the ears and over the natural 'brassiere'. With the pads of the fingers, use a circular action, completing each movement with an upwards sweep towards the chin. Do it every day; twice a day if your skin is dry or you work in a drying or polluted atmosphere.

Regular attention will clear away the dry, rough and leathery skin which accumulates at the base of the neck. Caring for this area also improves circulation and lymph drainage and strengthens the muscles which help to prevent sagging cheeks, jowls, jaw and chin. Those with problem skins will find that neck massage improves the blood supply to the face and speeds the healing of blemishes.

REHYDRATING WATER MIST

Spraying the neck and breasts with cold water after a moisturizing massage not only helps to tone muscle and improve circulation but also makes the moisturizer much more active and effective. Invest in an atomizer for this job and carry it with you as it's useful for 'setting' completed make-up, for freshening up during the day and for overcoming the negative effects of a very drying atmosphere. On a hot day, a facial spray is cooling and calming and provides instant relief to anyone suffering with those debilitating menopausal hot flushes.

If you have a refillable atomizer, mix mineral water with lavender essential oil (1fl oz/35ml water to 1 drop of oil) and spray the face regularly throughout the day, blotting excess away with tissues. Don't forget to close the eyes when spraying and remember to shake the container before each use.

WRINKLE REDUCER

Blend 6 drops of frankincense, 15 drops of lavender and 3 drops of neroli essential oil into 3fl oz/100ml of almond or olive oil. Massage a small amount *very gently* into those areas which are already wrinkled or where wrinkles are likely to form. Frankincense is believed to be able to help reduce existing wrinkles, lavender is balancing, calming and helps new cell growth and neroli helps to delay degeneration of cells and tissues.

VDU SCREENS

The air is full of electrically charged atoms. Outside, the fresh air consists mostly of beneficial negative ions. Inside buildings, especially those where there is much metal and electrical equipment, negative ions are often in short supply. The highly positive electrical charge which emanates from a VDU screen can change the polarity of the skin from its natural negative state to a positive one. Bacteria and viruses are then more likely to be attracted to the skin's surface, increasing the likelihood of spots, blemishes and, possibly, premature ageing.

Here's how to reduce the risk:

Take a ten-minute fresh air break every two hours. Go outside the building if possible – even on inclement, overcast days.
Find out if it is possible to open the windows.
Drink plenty of mineral water throughout the day.
Don't wear rubber- or plastic-soled shoes whilst sitting at your VDU.
Insist on the best quality filter for your screen.

Invest in an ionizer unit, which helps to increase the negative
    ions in the atmosphere.

Take plenty of exercise in the fresh air.

Take a daily antioxidant supplement (see pp.55–66, 73).

Practise deep breathing exercises every day (see p.190).

Rinse your face regularly throughout the day with fresh clean
    water, or spray with a water-filled atomizer, and reapply
    your moisturizer.

EYES RIGHT

The eyes are one part of the face which receives plenty of
attention but not necessarily the right treatment. We are
blessed with only one pair and yet we don't always look after
them well. These 'mirrors of the soul' are subjected to
squinting, bright lights, dust, smoke and make-up as well as
plenty of over-enthusiastic rubbing and pulling. Little wonder
that some of our first wrinkles appear underneath and at
either side of our eyes where the fine, thin skin is particularly
fragile.

Eye tissue contains very few oil glands and not that much
elasticity and so needs careful feeding. But never be tempted
to apply too much heavy cream in the belief that more is
better. The skin will soak it up – rather like a sponge full of
water, making the eyes puffy and sore. Use products which are
made specifically for the eyes. Apply and remove make-up
gently and never rub or stretch the skin.

There are several eye conditions, caused by a variety of factors,
which will often respond very favourably to simple dietary
changes. For example, there is evidence that cataracts can be

aggravated by a diet rich in dairy foods but low in antioxidant vitamins and minerals.

If you have smarting or itching eyes, are sensitive to light or have persistent redness in the whites of the eyes, you may benefit from an increase in wholegrain foods, less red meat, less milk, more fresh fish and more fresh fruit.

If your eye problems have occurred due to diabetes, your diet should be low in animal fats, rich in seeds, nuts, fruits, vegetables and fresh fish. Diabetics may also be unable to convert beta carotene, the vegetable source of vitamin A, into retinol (essential for eye health). A low-dose supplement of vitamin A in retinol form can be very beneficial in these circumstances.

Puffiness of the eyelids, protruding eyes or heavy bags under the eyes may be symptomatic of thyroid problems. Permanent dark circles can indicate poor digestion and food intolerance. Recurring conjunctivitis can often be related to poor immunity. Dry eyes and a lack of tear fluid suggests a deficiency of essential fatty acids; GLA or evening primrose oil supplements can help here.

Tired eyes will benefit from eye pads made of chamomile tea bags, cucumber slices or cotton pads soaked in herbal eyebright. Extract of angelica is an old herbal remedy used to soothe and repair the sensitive skin around the eye area and is now found in some quality eye creams.

Rest the eyes regularly throughout the day by palming. For two or three minutes at a time, sit in a comfortable chair and rest the elbows on a desk or table. With relaxed shoulders, place the hands over closed eyes and rock yourself gently backwards and forwards. Breathe deeply. This exercise is especially therapeutic for those working for long hours in front of a keyboard and VDU.

LIP SERVICE

The thinnest of skin covers the lips, which is why they are so prone to splitting and even bleeding. Always protect them with a special lip moisturizer; moisture-rich lipstick can also help. Cracks and chaps will benefit from gentle massage with the contents of a vitamin E capsule.

ON YOUR TOES

Feet walk an average of 115,000 miles in a lifetime. They support us and transport us. And yet the 26 bones, 33 joints, 10 nails and the skin which holds them all together are usually ignored. It is fact of life that improving foot care can enhance the health of the whole body.

So take a step in the right direction and cosset your hard-working feet each evening by soaking them in a relaxing footbath containing warm water and a few drops of essential oil, either stimulating peppermint, or lavender for relaxation. Then dry them thoroughly, rubbing briskly with a towel. Massage each foot with apricot or sesame seed oil, olive oil, peppermint foot cream or cocoa butter cream. Begin with the toes and use a gentle circular massage action over the whole foot including the toes, heels and ankles. It takes only a few minutes to nourish the feet in this way – and you moisturize your hands at the same time. Applying lubrication to the toes reduces the risk of nails growing inwards.

If your feet tend to perspire a lot, avoid using talcum powder; it collects around the nails, between the toes and in cracks and crevices and behaves rather like wet cotton wool, encouraging soreness and infection. If fungal infections of the foot are a problem, apply tea tree oil (or creams containing the oil) externally. In addition, take a six month course of acidophilus/bifidus supplements and remove all sugar and yeast from the diet.

Change socks and stockings daily. Don't wear the same pair of shoes every day. And choose a sensible heel height. Very flat shoes - as well as heels which are too high - can cause posture problems, back ache and spinal misalignment. Help tired feet by taking your shoes off during the day, wiggling your toes and rotating your ankles. Arnica cream helps to relieve the pain of bunions and stiff joints; juniper and lavender oils are also very soothing.

Keep toenails short; cut them straight across and never dig into the sides of the nail. If you suffer with corns, calluses or ingrowing toenails, don't try to deal with these problems yourself: consult a qualified chiropodist. A regular visit to a reflexologist is also highly recommended: this ancient healing art of foot massage can be beneficial for a variety of ailments, as well as being extremely relaxing.

FOUR

Well-Being

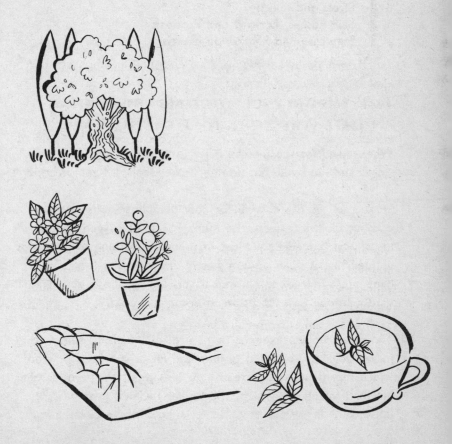

Breath of Life

The space between heaven and earth is like a bellows;
The shape changes but not the form;
The more it moves, the more it yields.
More words count less.
Hold fast to the centre.

Lao Tzu (?604–?531 BC), Tao Te Ching

> A Healing Power
> Inner Energy
> Stress and Toxicity
> Skin Rashes, Eczema and Psoriasis
> Breathing and Relaxation Exercises

THE IMPORTANCE OF DEEP BREATHING AND DE-STRESSING TO HEALTHY SKIN

When asked for the secret of her longevity (at age 80), the singer and vaudeville star Sophie Tucker replied 'Keep breathing'!

How true! We can survive for considerable periods of time without food, but starve the human body of oxygen and we die almost immediately. Most of us take breathing so much for granted that we can be completely unaware that it is happening; indeed, so ignored is this life-sustaining activity that hardly anyone pays attention to doing it properly.

The oldest known exercise or control of breathing comes from Indian yoga and is called pranayama. *Prana* is a Sanskrit word which means not only 'breath' but also refers to the underlying life force or energy which, the Indians believe, pervades the universe. It is the *Chi* or *Qi* of Oriental medicine. Hatha yoga,

chi gong, tai chi, meditation, rebirthing, massage and a host of
other therapies recognize the importance of breathing as a
healing power for the whole being and, particularly, as a way
to mend the mind.

The Chinese concept of health is that developing *Chi* to its full
potential will give abundant soundness, vigour, vitality and
longevity. If *Chi* decreases, body strength and inner energy
diminish also. The obstruction of this life force by poor
breathing, inadequate diet, an overactive mind, lack of exercise
and mental or emotional distress can result in the body
experiencing dis-ease.

To the Western world, unfamiliar with Oriental philosophy,
relaxing and resting the physical body doesn't always come
easily. In the quietest of rooms and the most peaceful of
surroundings, worry wanders in and out of the tranquillity and
overactive thoughts seem impossible to eradicate.

A tight throat, clenched jaw, hunched shoulders – even toes
gripped claw-like inside shoes – can be so familiar that such
mannerisms become part of the person who 'sets' into a rigid,
permanently stressed posture. As a result, physical tension is
placed upon organs, muscles and bones, particularly the neck,
spine and face.

Sadly, many over-stressed people accept their symptoms as a
normal part of everyday life and may not even be aware that
anything is wrong.

Prolonged and rapid shallow breathing – also known as
hyperventilation – means that oxygen and carbon dioxide are
exchanged inadequately. This can lead to dizziness, numbness,

confusion, poor co-ordination, muscle cramps, chest pain (often mistaken for heart problems), panic attacks and loss of perspective. And, to the great detriment of the skin and all its functions, toxicity! Decreased oxygen supply also *increases* hormone production from those probably already exhausted adrenal glands. Stress blocks the protective prostaglandins which, as well as performing many other jobs, help guard against viral invasion. Stress really can make you ill!

Watch someone breathing and, if you see any movement at all, it is often only the chest which rises and falls. The diaphragm and abdomen hardly move at all. Ask someone to indicate where in the body their lungs are positioned and they will usually point to the upper chest, forgetting - or perhaps, not even realizing - that these substantial breathing bags take up most of the space inside the rib cage. They fill the beehive-shaped area from just below the shoulders, all the way down to the curved diaphragm muscle spanning the base of the ribs - and from the spine at the back to the sternum at the front.

See checklist opposite to check your breathing habits.

Positive stress can be positively good for us. It acts as an incentive, an impetus which fuels our ambitions and motivates us towards further achievements. Spurred on by constructive stimulation, we can feel good and look good too. Like all emotions, the pleasure and equanimity of our attainments and accomplishments affect our whole being - and show most particularly in the face.

Excessive negative stress, on the other hand, is anathema to skin health.

Glance at this checklist; if you would answer 'yes' to most of these questions, then it may be time to slow down and learn some simple, easy-to-follow, deep breathing techniques. Your skin will certainly benefit.

Do you:

- Always feel tired during the day?
- Find it difficult to concentrate?
- Feel that your life moves at an uncontrollably frantic pace?
- Sleep badly or feel unrefreshed after a good night's rest?
- Seethe or suffer from boiling indignation for no apparently good reason?
- Worry about what other people think of you?
- Suffer from otherwise unexplained dizziness?
- Bite your nails or the skin around them?
- Feel restless when sitting still?
- Experience irregular heartbeats, palpitations, chest pain or tightness not associated with any medical condition?
- Suffer chest pain when anxious?
- Become breathless without exertion?
- Smoke or drink to calm your nerves?
- Suffer from attacks of panic?
- Take tranquilizers for a stress-related condition?
- Bottle up your emotions and find it difficult to express your feelings?
- Cry frequently or feel tearful?
- Feel stressed or 'wound up' without reason?

The term 'stress' has become the modern idiom for almost any problem related to mental and emotional overload. Sufferers – and those who live or work alongside them – cannot have failed to notice that pressure from persistent negative stress – and dis-stress – can also aggravate or be the cause of physical illness. A study carried out by the now defunct Common Cold Unit (reported in the *New England Journal of Medicine*) found that suffering negative stress nearly doubles the risk of 'catching' a cold. Cancer diagnoses can, all too frequently, be linked to traumatic life events which occurred 12 to 24 months before diagnosis. And no-one should be surprised. Where 20th-century pressures, pollution and poor eating habits collide with human animals who have evolved hardly at all since Palaeolithic times, there is bound to be inner conflict.

Until the horrors of Halcion (and other similar drugs) hit the headlines, prescribing tranquillizers and sleeping pills was the first line of treatment handed out by G.P.s.

Few doctors give diet a second thought when a patient presents a long list of seemingly unconnected symptoms. Add headaches to the list and painkillers are likely to be the order of the day.

If stress pushes up blood pressure, the patient may find him/herself on beta blockers, calcium antagonists, ACE inhibitors, vasodilators or thiazide diuretics. Stress-related indigestion may result in a further prescription for aluminium hydroxide antacids, sodium bicarbonate, proton pump inhibitors, H_2 blockers or reflux suppressants – to name but a few.

Skin rashes, urticaria (hives), eczema and psoriasis are often related to dietary difficulties, internal toxicity or a chronic anxiety state, but the medical answer is more likely to be a prescription for drugs or topical creams than a cleansing diet or a relaxation exercise. The patient has already embarked upon the downhill slope towards iatrogenic (doctor-induced) disease because of the negative side effects, the detrimental interactions of his drug cocktail and the reluctance or inability of his medical adviser to address the cause of his condition.

Modern day dis-stress is difficult to avoid. Unlike primitive man we neither run away from, nor face head on, the predators Fear and Anxiety which stalk us. Like a human pressure cooker, we avoid letting off steam to the point where we are under constant risk of exploding. The effect of this pent-up power puts an unhealthy strain upon all the body's organs. Hormonal glands over-secrete, nerves are 'on edge' and the stomach churns out excess acid. The digestive system shuts down, food is not broken down or absorbed properly, the body is undernourished and cannot repair and renew itself as it once did. High levels of stress are also likely to reduce levels of minerals such as iron, zinc, copper and selenium within the body. Under such circumstances, the skin is bound to suffer.

Deep sonorous breathing literally feeds the body and the brain. It calms an overactive mind, improves energy levels, reduces fatigue, lessens the risk of chest infections, improves the transport of oxygen and other vital nutrients around the body, enhances the quality of sleep and is particularly beneficial for improving cell turnover, for skin repair and condition. Correct breathing is a fundamental mechanism for attaining physical, mental, emotional and spiritual well-being. Learning the blessings and benefits of effective and efficient breathing is easy – and it's free!

The Basic Breathing Exercise

First of all, find out if you are a chest breather or a belly breather. Lie down on the bed. Place your right hand on your chest and your left hand on your abdomen. Breathe normally and notice which hand moves the most. If it is the right hand only, then you may not be breathing deeply enough.

Do the following exercise twice daily for ten 'in' breaths and ten 'out' breaths first thing in the morning before you get out of bed and last thing at night while you are waiting to go to sleep.

Try to ensure that your breathing cycle involves a slightly longer exhalation than inhalation, as this is believed to be important in reducing stress.

1. Lie on your back and make sure you are completely comfortable. Before you begin, be certain that you are relaxed, paying particular attention to those clenched toes, tight shoulders and clenched jaw!
2. Exhale gently and completely, drawing the abdomen inwards. Then, begin to breathe in so that your abdomen extends and the lower ribs expand ... keep in breathing in so that air fills your chest ... hold

A Simple Exercise to Quieten the Mind

1. Lie down in a warm, well-ventilated room.
2. Loosen any tight clothing.
3. Do your basic breathing exercise as usual.
4. Then make a picture in your mind of a hamster running around inside a wheel. This is your mind – racing.
5. Watch the hamster for a while. He is running so fast that you can't see clearly the rungs in his circular ladder.

for one second ... then exhale gently, emptying the air from the upper chest cavity and then from the abdomen. Hold for one second on the exhale before you start the next in-breath.

3. Your diaphragm should rise as you exhale and move downwards as you inhale. During the exercises, keep the mouth gently closed and breathe in and out through the nose. DO NOT STRAIN. Breathe to comfortable limits.

4. As you breathe out, imagine that you are pushing away all tension, anger, resentment, impatience and distress. As you breathe in, draw peace, tranquillity, warmth and comfort through the nose, into the lungs and into your body. Be aware of the coolness of the incoming air.

5. You may find it also helpful to picture breathing out darkness and breathing in white light.

6. Deep breathing helps to lower blood pressure. When you have completed your morning exercise, breathe normally for two minutes before getting out of bed. Ease yourself up very gently and sit on the side of the bed for 30 seconds or so before standing up.

Important Note: These breathing exercises are not suitable for anyone with a severe heart condition except under medical supervision.

---

6. Then see the wheel slowing down, slower and slower until it stops. You can picture the rungs in more detail.

7. The wheel stops going round.

8. The hamster is still there but he had turned over on to his back and is using the wheel as a hammock – rocking gently backwards and forwards.

9. After a while, the wheel stops moving altogether; all is quiet.

10. Finally, picture the hamster getting up out of the wheel and climbing into a huge cosy armchair. In a few moment, watch him fall fast asleep.

THE RELAXATION EXERCISE

This simple exercise can be carried out sitting in a straight-backed chair, or lying on one's back or one's side. It is said by the Chinese to be helpful for reducing lethargy and tension, stuffiness of the head and chest and also headaches.

1. Breathe normally and naturally through the nose with the tip of the tongue touching – gently – the roof of the mouth.
2. Breathe in and out twenty times, counting 'one' for each complete inhale and exhale.
3. Stop counting.
4. Let the tongue relax into its normal position and breathe normally.
5. Then THINK through your body, relaxing each section as you go. Work from the toes and feet upwards relaxing the legs, buttocks, abdomen, chest, arms, shoulders, neck, jaw, face and head.
6. Return to the feet and start again, this time making sure that the *right side* of the body is completely relaxed.
7. Then return again to the feet and relax the *left side*.
8. Lie or sit quietly for 10–15 minutes.

POLLUTION

Breathing in polluted air is an obvious hazard to health. We can't give up breathing but we can take precautions both to cut down the effects of pollution and to improve the strength and capacity of our lungs.

- If you go jogging, don't do it alongside heavy traffic.
- If you run or walk in a polluted area, invest in a mask. Cyclists wear them; why not pedestrians? The answer may be that people don't find them aesthetically pleasing to the eye. If the designers of high fashion designated protective masks as the latest accessory, our attitude towards them would doubtless change and the shops would run out of stock!
- If you are driving behind a smoky vehicle, temporarily shut off your own vehicle's incoming air. Better to breathe your own carbon dioxide for a few minutes than someone else's carbon monoxide.
- Daily deep breathing exercises indoors or away from polluted areas can help to eliminate accumulated toxins.
- Make sure your diet contains plenty of vitamin C-rich fruits, vegetables and salads.
- Take a gram (1000mg) tablet of vitamin C or antioxidant complex containing vitamin C every day.
- Fill your home and your workplace with anti-polluting green plants such as Cereus peruvianus, spider plant, chrysanthemum, peace lily or Chinese evergreen.

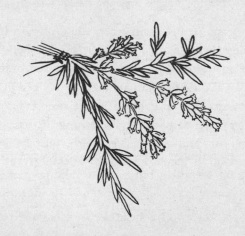

Sleep, Slumber
and Snooze

A good laugh and a long sleep are the best cures in the
doctor's book.

Old Irish proverb

Insomnia
Relaxation Tapes
Exercise
Essential Oils
Deep Breathing
Herbal Remedies

Getting a good night's sleep sounds simple and yet can be so
hard to achieve. Many things interrupt the best planned
slumbers: low blood sugar, nutrient deficiency (particularly of
minerals), noise, an unfamiliar room or bed, being too hot or
too cold, illness, pain, skin itching and irritation, an overactive
mind, excitement, anxiety, worry or depression.

The odd sleepless night can leave you feeling a bit jaded but is
unlikely detrimentally to affect your health. Long-term
insomnia, on the other hand, can lead to chronic exhaustion –
and it won't do anything beneficial for your skin, either. Lack
of sleep means that your brain is not rested. Fragmented sleep
does not give the same value as an uninterrupted seven or
eight hours and can lead to irritability, moodiness, poor
concentration, an increased risk of accidents and irrational
behaviour.

Some people will survive healthily and happily on as few as

three, four or five hours per night, their only worry being that they think they should be getting eight hours! But the body is clever and tends to take sleep when it needs it. Research shows that the majority of those who think they get very little sleep are in the Land of Nod for far longer than they imagine.

If you sleep for only a few hours but wake feeling rested, then you shouldn't concern yourself with trying to nap for longer. If you are a 'ten hours a night' person, that's fine too, as long as you don't wake up befuddled and sluggish.

If you are a long-term and natural insomniac but do not appear to be affected adversely, then settle for the number of hours you do sleep and make productive use of your waking time. If insomnia is something new, try some de-stressing techniques. Stress interferes with sleep more than almost anything else.

- Invest in a relaxation tape. Use it during the day or play it (on a machine which switches off automatically) while you are waiting to go to sleep.
- Set aside half an hour each day for rest and relaxation. Make yourself unavailable. The world won't stop turning as a result.
- Don't eat a heavy meal late at night and avoid stimulants (especially in the evening) such as coffee, tea, chocolate, salt, sugar, alcohol or nicotine.
- Take regular exercise during the day.
- Buy an oil burner and some lavender essential oil. Light the burner half an hour before bedtime so that aroma fills the room. Extinguish the light before retiring. Alternatively, you can buy small electric fans that blow air through essential oils; these can be left on without any worry (see Resources).
- Alternatively, put a few drops of lavender oil on a clean

tissue and pop it under your pillow. Herb-filled pillows may also be beneficial.

- Practise the deep breathing and relaxation exercises detailed in the chapter 'Breath of Life', p.196.
- Soak for ten minutes in a warm bath and then go straight to bed.
- Try yoga, tai chi or other meditation. Relaxing the mind during the day can mean that you need less sleep at night.
- Have regular aromatherapy or reflexology treatments – these help to release tension from the body and aid relaxation.
- Learn to catnap – and don't feel guilty about it. Our natural body clocks are designed for two sleeping periods in every 24 hours; one at night and another during the afternoon. Imagine how much less frantic the world would be if everyone went to sleep for an hour or two after lunch.
- If a particular worry is keeping you awake, ask yourself if that worry is productive and worthwhile. Usually it isn't.
- If you wake up during the night and can't get off to sleep again, don't lie there thrashing about. Read, listen to the radio or a tape – or get up and move around. Record a play from the radio and then listen to it in bed; you should drift off in no time.
- If hunger wakes you, it may be that your blood glucose levels have fallen too far. Try a small snack of cereal or yoghurt about an hour before bedtime.
- Don't resort to sleeping drugs except in extreme circumstances. They are toxic and can be addictive. Short-term use at times of severe distress and anxiety – such as bereavement for example – is entirely justified, but long-term popping of sleep-inducing medication is *not* recommended.
- Instead, try a herbal remedy which contains passiflora, valerian, skullcap, black cohosh and/or lady's slipper; or the calming minerals magnesium and calcium.

Exercise and Energize

Patients should have rest, food, fresh air and exercise – the quadrangle of health.

Sir William Osler (1849-1919), Canadian Physician

Gently Does It
Muscle Tone – and Skin Tone
Exercise Videos
Rebounding

Regular exercise can add life to your years by enhancing immune function, reducing cholesterol and blood pressure, increasing your 'staying power', developing muscle strength and lean body mass (to prevent sagging!), increasing oxygen uptake and lessening the risk of brittle bone disease. Daily activity also lifts mood, reduces anxiety and depression, dissolves negative stress, detoxifies the body and helps it to shed old and unwanted dead skin cells. Blood is drawn to the surface and nutrients are transported more efficiently around the system. Circulation and skin tone are improved.

But to achieve these benefits you don't need to climb Everest, run a marathon every day or work out to extremes. Strenuous over-exertion is likely to be just as detrimental to health as being a comatose couch potato. An increased risk of infections, hormonal imbalances, nutrient deficiencies and skeletal damage are all common to fitness freaks.

Gentle aerobics, keep fit classes, yoga, cycling, walking, dancing, sensible weight training, stretching and deep breathing are all beneficial types of exercise. Always make warm-up and wind-down movements part of your programme. If you want to work out to a home video, The Y Plan Countdown Video, Josh Salzmann's Bodyfit video or The Bodyplan Video are recommended (available from bookstores and video outlets).

Rebounding (on a mini-trampoline) for ten minutes a day can be as effective as half an hour pounding the tarmac – without weather problems or pollution and no need for specialist clothing (or high ceilings). Most good-quality rebounders come with a free exercise programme. (See Resources.)

Aim to exercise for 20 minutes a day or 45 minutes three times a week. Begin slowly at 5 minutes a day and increase gradually towards your target. Don't overdo it. Pushing yourself to the point where you are straining and out of breath means you are no longer working aerobically.

Important Note: Before embarking on any new exercise programme, seek out specialist assistance from a qualified fitness expert, aerobics teacher, swimming coach or gym instructor. If you have an existing health problem and are receiving medication, ask your practitioner for a health check.

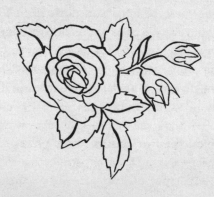

First Aid For Skin

Bites and stings
Brittle nails
Broken veins
Bumps and bruises
Burns
Chafing and chapped hands
Chilblains
Cracked lips
Cuts
Herpes
Itching
Scarring
Sore eyes
Sore throats
Spots and pimples
Sprains
Ulcers
Winter dryness

Quick-thinking and the application of first aid can make a huge difference in easing the pain of skin problems, from cracked lips and cold sores to insect bites and burns. First aid can also prevent a worsening of the condition and encourage rapid healing. It needn't be complicated - these treatments can be applied at home, often using ingredients from the kitchen cupboard such as tea bags, vegetable peelings, olive oil and honey. Herbal infusions, homoeopathic remedies and vitamin and mineral supplements also help to promote a speedy but gentle return to skin health.

Bites and Stings

If there is a sting remove it if possible and seek medical help if necessary. For wasp stings, pouring cider vinegar over the damaged area helps to draw the poison out, cleanse the wound and reduce the inflammation. For bee stings, apply bicarbonate of soda solution. And check with your G.P. as soon as possible; stings can cause unpleasant adverse reactions. Ant bites can be painful; apply crushed garlic or rub the sore area with cucumber skin. Take 2 grams of vitamin C every three hours and a daily B complex which contains B_5 and B_6 if you are bitten or stung: these nutrients have natural antihistamine properties and are good for distress. Also recommended are Homoeopathic Arnica and Bach Rescue Remedy for shock. Add tea tree oil or aloe vera juice to cooled boiled water to make an antiseptic wash. However, don't take tea tree oil internally or use it for stings inside the mouth. Homoeopathic Apis mellifica (Apis mel.) is helpful for stings which cause reddening, swelling and pain.

If you are visiting a mosquito-ridden area, swallow the equivalent of two fresh cloves of garlic every day, either raw, in cooking or as supplements. Mosquitoes and other biting insects hate the taste and smell and so are more likely to leave you alone. If you are attacked, bathe the bite with a soaked chamomile tea bag or rub with fresh elder leaves and crushed raw garlic. To relieve the itching caused by a mosquito bite, dissolve 2 teaspoons of baking powder in warm water and bathe the affected area or, alternatively, use a dilute solution of cider vinegar (one part vinegar to six parts water). Take a B complex (50mg three times a day) while you are exposed to mosquitoes. The essential oil citronella is a useful insect repellent, either applied with a carrier oil to the skin or used in an oil burner, especially during the night. Take artemesia (wormwood) herbal tablets for two weeks before travelling, continue during any visit abroad and use also as a treatment following mosquito attack. This medicine is proving beneficial in the treatment of malaria.

Brittle, Splitting and Flaking Nails

Massage the contents of a cod liver oil capsule and a vitamin E capsule into the nails every night (wear cotton gloves in bed if the smell or stickiness disturbs you) and take GLA or evening primrose oil supplements every day. See chapters 'Skin Nutrients' and 'Nails and Hands' (pp.55, 173).

Broken Veins

Damage to tiny capillaries occurs most commonly in areas where there is poor circulation and where thinner or ultra-sensitive skin is exposed to the atmosphere. They crop up when fragile capillary walls dilate and rupture, allowing blood to seep out into the tissues in minute quantities. The face and legs seem particularly susceptible. High blood pressure (hypertension) and some drug medicines, such as steroids and hydrocortisone creams, can aggravate the problem. (I was surprised to read recommendations by a skin-care expert who advised the use of such creams to *treat* broken veins - yet cortisone has a skin *thinning* effect.)

Sufferers should avoid very hot or very cold foods, spices, alcohol, salt, coffee and sugar. Increase your intake of fresh fruit - especially grapefruit, lemons, apples and avocados - and of raw beetroot, nuts, seeds, sprouted seeds and grains, eggs and cold-pressed oils. Supplement with beetroot extract (an excellent source of bioflavonoids which help to strengthen capillary walls), vitamin C (1000-2000mg daily) and vitamin E (100 - 400iu daily). Protect the skin against the drying effects of cold wind, central heating and air conditioning by always applying protective moisturizer and spraying the face regularly throughout the day with a water-mist. Some cosmetic companies produce very portable ready-to-use sprays made from mineral water and humectants - or you could refill your own atomizer with filtered or spring water.

Bumps and Bruises

Unless the skin is broken, rub the area gently but firmly for at least two minutes with the heel of your hand. This prevents the blood from blackening underneath the skin. Homoeopathic Arnica reduces the negative effects of trauma and the likelihood of bruising 'coming out'. Rub arnica cream or Derma C cream into the area three times each day for two or three days afterwards. And take vitamin C with bioflavonoids (1000mg three times daily) internally.

Burns

Hold the burnt area under a cold tap, or immerse in a bowl of iced water; keep immersed for as long as the pain continues. Then cover the area with cooled (cleaned and boiled) potato peelings and wrap with sterilized cotton cloth or bandages. Change the peelings twice daily. (Surgeons in Holland found this traditional method to be at least as good as current orthodox treatments.) Severe burns should receive immediate hospital attention (although first aid immersion in iced water still applies). Bach Rescue Remedy Cream, vitamin E cream or lavender oil are all soothing and healing to burned but unbroken skin. Taking vitamins A, C and E and zinc internally will hasten the healing of burns.

Chafing

Apricot and sesame seed oil are both excellent remedies for preventing the chafing caused by sports gear and new shoes. Cracked heels respond well to nightly massage with olive oil, cocoa butter or a nourishing foot cream.

Chapped Hands

Use a hand cream which contains vitamin E and/or aloe vera. Wear protective gloves for household jobs and always protect hands with mitts or gloves in cold weather. Take vitamin E and GLA or evening primrose oil every day, especially throughout the winter months. It also helps to pierce open a vitamin E and an evening primrose oil capsule, massaging the contents into your hands, nails and cuticles. Avoid sugar and sugary foods. Eat plenty of sunflower, pumpkin and linseeds.

Chilblains

An inflammation of the fingers or toes, usually due to poor circulation and inadequate nutrition. Help to strengthen blood vessels by taking a regular vitamin C complex and/or a bioflavonoid supplement such as the new Beetroot Concentrate. Freshly juiced raw beetroot is helpful for the blood and circulation too. Eat more dark green vegetables and fresh fruits, live yoghurt, nuts and seeds. Vitamin E (100-400iu daily) and GLA or evening primrose oil capsules are a wonderful boost to a sluggish circulation. Homoeopathic Silica is another useful remedy. Massage painful chilblains with marigold, calendula or arnica cream.

Cracked Lips

Lips crack very easily because the skin covering them is very thin and has no moisturizing oil supply of its own. Use Bach Rescue Remedy Cream daily under lipstick or by itself to lubricate dry lips and apply a protective coat of the same cream before bedtime. When using facial scrubs, exfoliate gently over and around the lip area to remove any dead skin.

Cuts

Superficial cuts will heal more quickly if bathed in aloe vera juice. Six drops of tincture of myrrh in warm water is a useful mixture for cleansing dirty wounds. If the cut is deep, seek medical help. Once a cut has closed up and is beginning to heal, rub it daily with the contents of a vitamin E capsule to prevent scarring.

Herpes

Herpes is a highly contagious viral condition; once the virus has taken up residence in the body, it can lie dormant for years but will never go away. However, if treated correctly, it *is* controllable. There are many kinds of herpes which fall into two distinct groups.

Herpes simplex is an inflammatory skin condition characterized by the formation of small clusters of watery blisters. Cold sores (*herpes labialis*) belong to this 'family' as does *herpes genitalis* which affects the mucous membranes of the genitalia. Both are highly contagious and can be passed from one part of the body to another by touch. It is imperative to be cautious during an attack of herpes because of its transferable characteristics. The virus can be passed easily by kissing. This kind of herpes is a sexually transmittable disease; intimate contact during an attack is obviously not recommended. Unfortunately, however, symptoms are not always visible and may take several weeks to appear – if at all. If you do suspect herpes infection, it is imperative that you see your G.P. without delay.

Herpes zoster (shingles) is an acute inflammatory condition triggered by the same virus that causes chicken-pox and which affects the nervous system. Pain during an attack can be very severe indeed and is often followed by a post-herpetic neuralgia.

Medical treatment of herpes with antiviral drugs can be very effective; but supporting the immune system and managing stress are also key factors in the control and prevention of herpes. It is also believed to have a hormonal connection since flare-ups do sometimes happen during periods.

Improving the quality of the diet and taking regular supplements can boost the immunity, strengthen stress resistance and help to balance hormones. I have found particular success in treating patients with short-term cleansing diets (3 or 4 days) of fresh fruits, vegetables, salads and water followed by sugar-free, additive-free wholefoods, fresh fish, live yoghurt and lots of fresh produce – organic if possible. Herpes sufferers should avoid stimulants such as alcohol, salt, sugar, nicotine and caffeine.

If you have herpes and would like to try using nutritional supplements to ease your condition, these are the ones which I have found most helpful with my own patients.

- A multivitamin/mineral complex which contains vitamins A, E, B$_6$ and zinc (one daily).
- Vitamin B$_{12}$ (injections once monthly for three months from your GP, or a three-month supply of enteric-coated tablets, one daily). Vitamin B$_{12}$ is the anti-pernicious anaemia vitamin but also has a major role to play in the function of a healthy nervous system, proving useful in the treatment of a range of neurological conditions.
- Two grams of vitamin C complex daily. Vitamin C is naturally anti-viral, helps boost immunity and has natural painkilling activity.
- Free form amino acid powders containing lysine, which is well known for the amelioration of herpes. This product is expensive, and *should be taken only under practitioner supervision*.
- *Lactobacillus acidophilus* probiotic supplements help to improve the quality of friendly bacteria in the gut and to boost immunity. In addition, probiotics have an oestrogen-balancing activity which may be a helpful addition in the treatment of herpes.
- Bioflavonoid Complex. Bioflavonoids help to reduce inflammation and are also powerful antioxidants. See page 62 and Resources.
- Vitamin E is useful for both topical and oral treatment of herpes. Take 400–600iu daily with meals and in addition apply the contents of one or two capsules to the affected areas. Remember to wash the hands thoroughly after application. Vitamin E acts to reduce inflammation and, as a result, may also reduce pain. It has been used very successfully in the treatment of neuralgia pain associated with herpes zoster.
- Tea tree oil; see page 147. Wash the hands thoroughly afterwards.

Itchy Skin

Can be caused by a disturbed pH balance. Try putting a tablespoon of extra virgin olive oil and two tablespoons of organic cider vinegar (not malt or wine vinegar) in the bath water. Very soothing too for psoriasis, eczema and dermatitis and for that most embarrassing and distressing of 'itches', pruritis.

Scarring

To reduce the risk of scars forming (after accident or surgery) and to help fade old scars, rub the oil from a vitamin E capsule gently but firmly into the traumatized area every night before bedtime. Derma C is also useful.

Sore Eyes

Bathe with a dilute witch hazel or eyebright solution. Herbal eyebright tablets are also available from most health food stores. Rest quietly in a darkened room with the eyes gently (not tightly) closed for 15 minutes during the day. Used, cold tea bags – one over each eye – reduce redness, puffiness and that gritty feeling. Take an antioxidant complex daily.

Sore Throats

Put two teaspoons of organic cider vinegar and one teaspoon of good-quality liquid honey into a cup or mug; top up with boiling water and then wait for it to cool to a comfortable temperature. Gargle until all the mixture has been used, swallowing each mouthful as you go. Repeat the process five or six times each day but especially first thing in the morning and last thing at night. Continue with the gargle for a couple of days after symptoms have subsided. Use the whole drink at each session and make a fresh batch each time. The honey soothes whilst the cider vinegar kills bacteria.

Spots and Pimples

Golden Seal herbal infusion used as a skin rinse is soothing and healing. Self-disinfecting 'spot' pens are also useful for emergency treatment, but beware of those which have too strong an alcohol base as they can be harsh and over-drying. Those based on active essential oils seem to be the most successful. (See Resources for further information).

Sprains

To bring down swelling, make a cold compress with diluted witch hazel, cold, used tea bags or ice cubes. Massage gently with transdermal C ointment, arnica or calendula ointment.

Ulcers

Any ulceration of the mucous membrane, whether it be in the mouth, the stomach or the small intestines, can be caused by nutrient deficiency coupled to poor digestion and irritation or infection. Freshly juiced vegetables and diluted fresh fruit juices (taken separately from other foods) can be most beneficial. Or try drinking the water that would normally be thrown away after cooking vegetables. Cabbage water is an age-old remedy for ulcers and contains a relatively unknown healing nutrient called vitamin U, which is also available in specialized supplement form. Also helpful are capsules of B complex, zinc, vitamin A, beta carotene and liquorice. Sage and calendula or aloe vera mouthwash is soothing and healing. Tincture of myrrh is an effective remedy for dabbing directly on to mouth ulcers or for use as a mouthwash: add 3ml of the tincture to a glass of water and use four times daily.

Wind, Winter and Central Heating Dryness

Restore the skin's protective acid mantle by rinsing with organic cider vinegar, either diluted and splashed over the skin or applied with cotton wool. Watch out for sudden and frequent changes of temperature. Stuffy, overheated offices to chilling outdoor winds and back again can make skin dry, sore and prone to broken veins. So, too, can drying summer wind and over-exposure to UV rays. In drying conditions, moisture is lost from the skin faster than it can be replaced, so make regular daily use of the water-mist spray mentioned above. Where broken thread veins are visible, massage the area very gently each night with the contents of a vitamin E capsule. Don't forget that bioflavonoids are helpful for this condition.

Recommended Reading

Ageless Ageing by Leslie Kenton, Century Arrow 1985

The Allergy Survival Guide by Jane Houlton, Vermillion 1993

Aromatherapy – A Guide For Home Use by Christine Westwood, Amberwood Publishing Ltd., Mulberry Court, Stour Road, Christchurch, Dorset BH23 1PS, England 1991

Aromatherapy, An A–Z by Patricia Davies, The C.W. Daniel Company Ltd., 1 Church Path, Saffron Walden, Essex CB10 1JP, England 1988

The Aromatherapy Handbook by Daniele Ryman, The C.W. Daniel Company Ltd., 1984

Candida Albicans Special Diet Cookbook by Richard Turner and Elizabeth Simonsen, Thorsons 1989

Candida Albicans – Yeast and Your Health by Gill Jacobs, Optima 1990

Cellulite Revolution by Leslie Kenton, Ebury Press 1992

Endless Energy by Susannah and Leslie Kenton, Vermillion 1993

The Food Combining Diet by Kathryn Marsden, Thorsons 1993

How to Ease Your Child's Eczema Without Drugs by Charles Lee. Available from The Allergy Shop Ltd., P.O. Box 196, Haywards Heath, West Sussex RH16 3YF, England.

Juicing for Health by Caroline Wheater, Thorsons 1993

The Natural Beauty Book by Anita Guyton, Thorsons 1991

A New Way of Eating by Marilyn Diamond, Bantam Books 1987

Save Your Skin With Vital Oils by Liz Earle, Vermillion/Ebury Press 1992

Self-Massage by Jacqueline Young, Thorsons 1992

Super Healthy Hair, Skin and Nails by Stella Weller, Thorsons 1991

10 Day Clean-Up Plan by Leslie Kenton, Century 1986

Zone Therapy by Joseph Corvo, Vermillion/Arrow 1993

References

References are listed according to order of discussion within the text.

Fat Facts, pp. 41-54

5th International Colloquium on Mono-unsaturated Fatty Acids. 17 and 18 February 1992.

Isles C.G., Hole D.J., Gillis C.R. et al. 'Plasma cholesterol, coronary heart disease and cancer'. Br.Med.J. 1989; 298:920-24.

Dietary Reference Values for Food Energy and Nutrients for the United Kingdom. Report of the Panel on Dietary Reference Values of the Committee on Medical Aspects of Food Policy.

Mensink R.P., Katan M.B. 'Effect of a diet enriched with monounsaturated or polyunsaturated fatty acids on levels of low-density lipoprotein cholesterol in healthy men and women'. N.Eng.J.Med 1989; 321(7):436-41.

Holborow P. 'Melanoma patients consume more polyunsaturated fat than people without melanoma'. N.Z. Med J. 27.11.91 p.502.

Report by Sir John McMichael. Br.Med.J. January 1979.

Halliwell B. Free Radicals and Food Additives. Pub. Taylor & Francis 1991.

Lipids in Human Nutrition by Professor G.J. Brisson.

Nutrition Against Disease by Dr Roger Williams.

Antioxidant Vitamins and Beta Carotene in Disease Prevention International Conference. October 1989.

Clausen J., Nielsen S.A., Kristensen M. 'Biochemical and clinical effects of an anti-oxidative supplementation of geriatric patients'. Biological Trace Element Research. 1989; 20:135-51.

Chow G.K. 'Nutritional influence on cellular antioxidant defence systems'. American Journal of Clinical Nutrition. 1979; 32:1066-81.

Gutteridge J.M., Westermarck T., Halliwell B. 'Oxygen radical damage in biological systems'. Free Radicals, Ageing and Degenerative Disease. 1986; pp.99-139.

Ito N., Hirose M. Antioxidants - carcinogenic and chemopreventive properties. 1989; 53:247-302.

Skin Nutrients, pp. 55-88

Okita M. et al. 'Lipid malnutrition of patients with liver cirrhosis; effect of low intake of dietary lipid on plasma fatty acid composition.' Acta Med Okayama. 1989; 43:39-45.

Zurer B. 'Essential fatty acids and inflammation'. Ann Rheum Dis. 1991; 50:745-46.

Holborow P. 'Melanoma and fatty acids'. NZ Med J. 1991; 104:19.

Begin M. et al. 'Plasma fatty acid levels in patients with Acquired Immune Deficiency Syndrome and in controls'. Prostaglandins Leukotr EFAs. 1989; 37:135-37.

Williams L.L. et al. 'Serum fatty acid composition of plasma from AIDS patients and normal individuals'. Arch AIDS RES. 1988; 23:981-88.

Manku M., Horrobin D.F., Morse N.L. et al. 'Essential fatty acids in the plasma phospholipids of patients with atopic eczema'. Br J Dermatol. 1984; 110:643-48.

Horrobin D.F. 'Essential fatty acids, immunity and viral infections'. J Nutr Med. 1990; 1:145-51.

Horrobin D.F. 'Essential fatty acids and the post-viral fatigue syndrome'. Book: Post Viral Fatigue Syndrome. Ed. Jenkins R. and Mowbray J. John Wiley, Chichester and New York 1991.

Wolfe S.M. *Pills That Don't Work*, pp. 18-19. Public Citizen Research Group.

Colbin A. *Food and Healing*, pp. 15-23. Ballantine Books.

Medawar C. *The Wrong Kind of Medicine*. Consumers' Association/Hodder & Stoughton, August 1984.

Coutsoudis A., Coovadia H.M., Broughton M., Salisbury R.T., Elson I.'Micronutrient utilization during measles treated with vitamin A or placebo'. *Int J Vitamin Nutrition Review*. 1991; 61:199-204.

Daulaire N. et al. 'Childhood mortality after a high dose of vitamin A in a high risk population'. *Br.Med.J.* 1992; 304:207-10.

Zile M.H., Cullum M.E. 'The function of vitamin A - current concepts'. *Proceedings of the Society of Experimental Biological Medicine*. 1983; 172:139-52.

Horwitt M.K. 'Data supporting supplementation of humans with vitamin E'. *J Nutr.* 1991; 121:424-29.

Janero D.R. 'Therapeutic potential of vitamin E in the pathogenesis of spontaneous atherosclerosis'. *Free Radical Biology & Medicine*. 1991; 11:129-44.

Marsden K. 'Vitamin C, the master nutrient versus heart disease, the master killer'. (article) *Int. J. Alt. Comp. Med.* October 1992 pp. 19-20.

Pauling L., Rath M. 'Solution to the puzzle of human cardiovascular disease'. *J Orthomolecular Med.* 1991; 6:125-34.

Ginter E. 'Vitamin C deficiency, cholesterol metabolism and atherosclerosis'. *J Orthomolecular Med.* 1991; 6:166-72.

Vitamin C - The Master Nutrient by Sandra Goodman. Published by Keats Publishing Inc.

Ginter E., Bobek P., Kubec F., Vozar J. Urbanova D. 'Vitamin C in the control of hypercholesterolaemia in man'. *International Journal of Vitamin and Nutritional Research*. 1982; 23:137-52.

Gorrie D.R. 'Purpura haemorrhagica after arsenic therapy treated by vitamin P'. *Lancet*. 1940; 1:1005-7.

Middleton E. et al. 'Naturally occurring flavonoids and human basophil histamine release'. *Archives of Allergy & Applied Immunology*. 1985; 77:155-57.

Rixier J.M., Godeau G., Robert A.M. and Hornebeck W. 'In vivo and in vitro study demonstrating that binding of Pycnogenol to elastin affects its rate of degradation'. *Biochem.Pharmacol.* 1984; 33(24):3933-39.

Havsteen B. 'Flavonoids, a class of natural products of high pharmacological potency'. Article. *Biochem.Pharmacol.* 1983; 32(7):1141-48.

Ginter E. 'Vitamin C deficiency, cholesterol metabolism and atherosclerosis'. *J Orthomolecular Med.* 1991; 6:166-72.

Roediger W.E.W., Lawson M.J., Radcliffe B.C. 'Nitrite from inflammatory cells - a cancer risk factor in ulcerative colitis?' *Dis Colon Rectum*. 1990; 33:1034-36.

Tanji J.L. 'Dietary calcium as a treatment for mild hypertension'. *J Amer Board Family Practice*. 1991; 4:145-50.

Lipkin M. 'Calcium, vitamin D and colon cancer'. *Cancer Res*. 1991; 51:3069-70.

Bachert C. et al. 'Decreased reactivity in allergic rhinitis after intravenous application of calcium. A study on the alteration of local airway resistance after nasal allergen provocation'. *Arzneimittelforsch.*(translation) 1990; 40:984-87.

Anderson R.A. et al. 'Supplemental chromium effects on glucose, insulin, glucagon and urinary chromium losses in subjects consuming low chromium diets'. *Am J Clin Nutr.* 1991; 54:909-16.

Roeback J. 'Effect of chromium supplementation on serum high-density lipoprotein cholesterol levels in men taking beta-blockers'. *Ann Int Med.* 1991; 115(12):917-24.

Barber S.A., Bull N.L. and Buss D.H. 'Low Iron Intake Among Young Women in Britain.' *Br.Med.J.* 1985; 290:743-44

Woods K.L., Fletcher S., Roffe C., Haider Y. 'Intravenous magnesium sulphate in suspected acute myocardial infarction: results of second Leicester Intravenous Magnesium Intervention Trial'. *Lancet*. 1992; 39:1553-58.

Facchinetti F. et al. 'Oral magnesium successfully relieves premenstrual mood changes'. *Obstet Gyn.* 1991; 78:177-81.

Peretz A. et al. 'Adjuvant treatment of recent onset rheumatoid arthritis by selenium supplementation'. *Br J Rheumatol.* 1992; 31:281-86.

Abraham G.E. 'The importance of magnesium in the management of primary osteoporosis'. *J Nutr Med.* 1991; 2:165-78.

Acne Attack, pp.136-149

Bassett I.B., Pannowitz D.L. and Barnetson R.S.C. 'A comparative study of tea-tree oil versus benzoyl peroxide in the treatment of acne'. *Med.J.Australia* 1990; 153:455-58.

Eczema and Psoriasis, pp.150-163

Manku M.S., Horrobin D.F., Morse N.L., Wright S. and Burton J.L. 'Essential fatty acids in the plasma phospholipids of patients with atopic eczema'. *British Journal of Dermatology* 1984; 110:643-48.

Ziboh V.A. and Chapkin R.S. 'Metabolism and function of skin lipids'. *Progress in Lipid Research* 1988; 27:81-105.

Burton J.L. 'Dietary fatty acids and inflammatory skin disease'. *Lancet* 7.1.89; 27-30.

Vahlquist C. et al. 'The fatty acid spectrum in plasma and adipose tissue in patients with psoriasis'. *Archives of Dermatological Research* 1985; 278:114-19.

Maurice P. et al. 'The effects of dietary supplementation with fish oil in patients with psoriasis'. *British Journal of Dermatology* 1987; 177:599-606.

Stewart J.C. 'Treatment of severe and moderately severe atopic dermatitis with evening primrose oil'. *Journal of Nutritional Medicine* 1991; 2:9-15.

Sampson H. 'Role of immediate food hypersensitivity in the pathogenesis of atopic dermatitis'. *J. Allergy Clin.Immunology* 1983; 71:473-80.

Amella M. et al. 'Inhibition of mast cell histamine release by flavonoids and bioflavonoids'. *Planta Medica* 1985; 51:16-20.

Sleep, Slumber and Snooze, pp.200-202

Penland J. 'Effects of trace element nutrition on sleep patterns in adult women'. *Federation of America Society of Experimental Biology Journal.* 1988; 2:434.

Exercise and Energize, pp.203-213

McGuire R. 'Twice daily exercise may reduce hypertension'. *Medical Tribune* 27 June 1991.

Blair S.N., Goodyear N.N., Gibbons L.W. et al. 'Physical fitness and incidence of hypertension in healthy normotensive men and women'. *Ann.Rev.Public Health* 1987; 252:480-87.

Leon A.S., Connett J., Jacobs D.R. et al. 'Leisure-time physical activity levels and risk of coronary heart disease and death. The Multiple Risk Factor International Trial'. *J.Am.Med.Assoc.* 1987; 258:2388-95.

Duncan J.J. et al. 'Women Walking For Health And Fitness: How Much Is Enough?' *J.Am.Med.Assoc.* 1991; 266 (23):3295-99.

Frankel T. 'Walking may protect hips'. *Prevention magazine* 8 February 1990.

Lennox S.S., Bedell F.R., Stone A.A.. 'The effect of exercise on normal mood'. *J.Psychosomatic Res.* 1990; 34(6):629-636.

Braverman E.R. 'Sports and Exercise: Nutritional Augmentation and Health Benefits'. *J.Orthom.Med.* 1991; 6:191-201.

Caren L.D. 'Effects of exercise on the human immune system: does exercise influence susceptibility to infections?' *Bioscience* 1991; 41:410-15.

McLellan R. Article on rebounding. *The American Chiropractor,* June 1991 pp.10-14.

Resources

When writing to any of these addresses, please enclose a large stamped addressed envelope or international reply coupons.

Xynergy aloe vera juice and gel

Biogenic Aloe Juice for internal use. Aloe 99 Gel for external treatment of bites, stings, bruises, bedsores, burns etc. *Very highly recommended*. Available from good health stores. For stockist details, contact:

Xynergy Health Products, Lower Elsted, Midhurst, West Sussex GU29 0JT. Telephone: 01730. 813642.

Arbonne International

Swiss skin care products via mail order and through local consultants. For brochure and product details call:

Arbonne UK Ltd., Maids Moreton House, Buckingham MK18 1SW. Telephone: 01280. 824599.

Samuel Par

Specialist products for acne and oily skin made from natural plant extracts and essential oils. Highly recommended. Contact for stockist details:

UK – Bioconcepts Ltd., 6–10 Road View, Rudmore, Portsmouth, Hampshire PO2 8DT. Telephone: 01705.678131

USA – The Bailey Group, 7760 Romaine Street, West Hollywood, 90046 California. Telephone: 213.654.3301.

France – Samuel Par, 46 rue Madame, 75006 Paris. Telephone: 47.27.55.80.

Biocare

Vitamins and minerals including antioxidants, probiotics, linseed oil, Iron EAP2, Derma C cream, Artemesia Complex, chromium and G.L.A. Excellent quality and reliability.

Biocare Ltd., Lakeside, 180 Lifford Lane, Kings Norton, Birmingham B30 3NT. Telephone: 0121. 433.3727.

Blackmores

Skin care products, herbals, minerals and antioxidant supplements.

Blackmores UK – the Naturopathic Health & Beauty Co. Ltd., 37 Rothschild Road, Chiswick, London W4.

Australia: Blackmores, 23 Roseberry Street, Balgowlah 2093, New South Wales, Australia. Telephone: (02).949.3177.

Pharma Nord

Antioxidant, Co-enzyme Q10 and G.L.A. supplements. For stockist information contact:

Pharma Nord (UK) Ltd., Spital Hall, Mitford, Morpeth, Northumberland NE61 3PN. Telephone: 01670.519989.

Aromatherapy Oils and Related Products

Nelson's Pharmacy, 73 Duke Street, Grosvenor Square, London W1M 6BY. Telephone: 0171. 495.2404.

Also:
Gerard House, 475 Capability Green, Luton, Bedfordshire LU1 3LU. Telephone: 01582. 487331.

Water Filter Products

Available from most good hardware stores, health food shops and chemists.

Juicing Equipment

From stores supplying electrical goods. In case of difficulty call Kenwood on 01705.476000.

Non-hydrogenated Spreads such as Vitaquell

Available from most health food stores.

UK Distributors: Brewhurst Health Food Supplies, Abbot Close, Oyster Lane, Byfleet, Surrey KT14 7JP. Telephone: 01932.354211.

Organic Food Supplies

The Soil Association, 86 Colston Street, Bristol, Avon BS1 5BB. Telephone: 0272.290661. They will provide Regional Guides giving information relating to stockists, opening times, types of produce sold, delivery and mail order services county by county.

Amway

Suppliers of rebounders and also biodegradeable household products. For details of nearest distributor, write to:

Amway Information Centre, Snowdon Drive, Winterhill, Milton Keynes, Bucks. MK6 1AR. Telephone: 01908.691588. Amway products are available worldwide.

BUAV

Guide to cosmetics, household products and toiletries which have not been tested on animals.

British Union for the Abolition of Vivisection (BUAV), 16a Crane Grove, London N7 8LB. Please send a large s.a.e.

Berrydales

Provide valuable information for allergy sufferers. Regular newsletter, special diet cookbook, nutrition news and product info. Contact them at: 5 Lawn Road, London NW3 2XS. Telephone: 0171.722.2866.

Organic Honey and Tea Tree Oil Products

New Zealand Natural Food Company, Unit 7, 55–57 Park Royal Road, London NW10 7JP. Telephone: 0181.961.4410.

Revital Mail Order Service

Wide range of quality branded products including supplements, homoeopathic medicines, herbs, colon care, skin care. Contact:

Revital, 35 High Road, Willesdon, London NW19 2TE. Telephone: 0181.459.3382. Fax: 0181.459. 3722

or
Revital, 3a The Colonnades, 123/151 Buckingham Palace Road, London SW1W 9RZ. Telephone: 0171.976.6615 Fax: 0171.976.5529.

Kitchen Utensils, Equipment and Household Items

For catalogue containing a wide variety of practical utensils:

Lakeland Plastics, The Creative Kitchenware Company, Alexandra Buildings, Windermere, Cumbria LA23 1BQ. Telephone: 015394.88100.

Specialist Suppliers of Foods

Ideal for those with skin problems, food intolerances and allergic reactions:

Complementary Medicine Services, 9 Corporation Street, Taunton, Somerset TA1 4AJ. Allergy Care brochure. Telephone 'advice desk': 01823. 325022. Telephone orders: 01823.321027.

Organic Chocolate

Available in most major supermarkets. In case of difficulty, contact:

Green & Black, P.O. Box 1937, London W11 1ZU. Telephone: 0171.243.0562 or 0171.229. 7545.

Tea and Coffee

Better quality teas and coffees tend to be naturally lower in caffeine without the need to use decaffeinated products. For information, price list and mail order supplies, contact:

Kendricks Coffee Company, Tea and Coffee Specialists, Ocean Parade, South Ferring, Worthing, West Sussex BN12 5QQ. Telephone: 01903.503244.

The Women's Environmental Network

For those interested in keeping up to date with environmental issues. Send large stamped addressed envelope for details. Membership available.

The Women's Environmental Network, Aberdeen Studios, 22 Highbury Grove, London, N5 2EA. Telephone: 0171.354.8823.

Homoeopathic Medicines

Available from health food stores and by mail from: Ainsworths Homoeopathic Pharmacy, 38 New Cavendish Street, London W1M 9FG. Telephone: 0171.935.5330.

How to Find a Practitioner

If you live in London, the following multi-therapy centres have a staff of qualified practitioners and offer a wide range of services and valuable information:

All Hallows House, Centre for Natural Health, Idol Lane, London EC3R 5DD. Telephone: 0171.283. 8908, Monday to Thursday.
Nutrition therapy, McTimoney chiropractic, acupuncture, homoeopathy etc.

If you are outside London, All Hallows will try to help you find a practitioner nearer to your home. For their Candida directory and information pack – which gives details of therapists around the UK who specialize in the treatment of candidiasis – please send a large stamped addressed envelope to All Hallows House.

The following UK-based organisations hold lists of registered practitioners. If you write, please send a stamped addressed envelope:

The McTimoney Chiropractic Association, 21 High Street, Eynsham, Oxford OX8 1HE. Telephone: 01865.880974. For information on McTimoney training courses, contact The McTimoney Chiropractic School, 14 Park End Street, Oxford OX1 1HH. Telephone: 01865.246786.

The British Chiropractic Association, 29 Whitley Street, Reading, Berkshire RG2 0EG. Telephone: 01734.757557.

Candida – see All Hallows House (above).

The Institute for Complementary Medicine (ICM), P.O. Box 194, London SE16 1QZ. Telephone: 0171.237.5175.

The National Federation of Spiritual Healers, will provide you with the name of a healer in your area. Call them on 01891.616080.

The UK Homoeopathic Medical Association, 6 Livingston Road, Gravesend, Kent DA12 5DZ.

Colonic International Association, 31 Eton Hall, Eton College Road, London NW3 2DE.

British Complementary Medicine Association, St. Charles Hospital, Exmoor Street, London W10 6DZ.

Tests

For nutritional deficiencies, food allergies, intestinal parasites, full blood profile, contact:.

Biolab, 9 Weymouth Street, London W1N 3FF. Your doctor can contact them on 0171.636. 5905/5959.

Note: The following are available from health food stores and/or chemists: olive oil cream; skin brushes; loofah mitts; rescue cream; Bach Flower Remedies; Lecithin; linseeds; extra virgin olive oil; organic cider vinegar; gluten free products.

Index